Welcome to the EVERYTHING® series!

These handy, accessible books give you all you need to tackle a difficult project, gain a new hobby, comprehend a fascinating topic, prepare for an exam, or even brush up on something you learned back in school but have since forgotten.

You can read an *EVERYTHING*® book from cover to cover or just pick out the information you want from our four useful boxes: e-facts, e-ssentials, e-alerts, and e questions. We literally give you everything you need to know on the subject, but throw in a lot of fun stuff along the way, too.

We now have well over 100 *EVERYTHING*® books in print, spanning such wide-ranging topics as weddings, pregnancy, wine, learning guitar, one-pot cooking, managing people, and so much more. When you're done reading them all, you can finally say you know *EVERYTHING*®!

FACTS

Important sound bytes of information

SSENTIALS

Quick handy tips

ALERT

Urgent warnings

QUESTIONS?

Solutions to common problems

THE
EVERYTHING
Series®

Dear Reader,
Welcome to *The Everything® Menopause Book*—and join the crowd! More women are preparing to enter menopause now than at any time in history. Over 21 million American women are in menopause "countdown," and every day nearly 5,000 enter menopause. And this is one lucky bunch of women, too. Today, we know more about the physical and emotional symptoms of menopause than at any time in our past, and we have not only more effective treatment options but also more treatment options available to help make the menopause transition a healthy, smooth passage into the next phase of life.

Lots of information about menopause is available today, and much of it is confusing, contradictory, and hard to track down—and some of it is just plain wrong. We've prepared a concise, enjoyable, easy-to-read guide to menopause that lays out the facts—the information you need to make important decisions about your health and well-being through menopause and beyond. We've tried to present an unbiased view of menopause treatment options, using the most up-to-date, scientific data available. We've also tried to eliminate some of the confusion surrounding controversial topics. We encourage you to keep an open mind as you read through the book, because every menopause dilemma has a number of practical solutions.

You won't find some things in here, though; we've left out the fluff, the condescending patter, the confusing double-talk, and the well-honed sales pitches. What's left is just good, solid, practical information presented in a no-nonsense, jargon-free "read." We hope you enjoy reading *The Everything®* *Menopause Book* as much as we enjoyed writing it.

THE
EVERYTHING®
MENOPAUSE
BOOK

Reassuring advice and the
latest information to keep
you healthy and sane

Ramona Slupik, M.D., F.A.C.O.G.,
with Lorna Gentry

Adams Media Corporation
Avon, Massachusetts

EDITORIAL

Publishing Director: Gary M. Krebs

Managing Editor: Kate McBride

Copy Chief: Laura MacLaughlin

Acquisitions Editors: Bethany Brown,
Allison Carpenter Yoder

Development Editor: Michael Paydos

Production Editor: Khrysti Nazzaro

PRODUCTION

Production Director: Susan Beale

Production Manager: Michelle Roy Kelly

Series Designer: Daria Perreault

Cover Design: Paul Beatrice and Frank Rivera

Layout and Graphics: Colleen Cunningham,
Rachael Eiben, Michelle Roy Kelly,
Daria Perreault, Erin Ring

An Everything® Series Book.
Everything® is a registered trademark of Adams Media Corporation.

Published by Adams Media Corporation
57 Littlefield Street, Avon, MA 02322 U.S.A.
www.adamsmedia.com

ISBN: 1-58062-741-2
Printed in the United States of America.

J I H G F E D C B A

Library of Congress Cataloging-in-Publication Data
Gentry, Lorna.
The everything menopause book / Lorna Gentry, Ramona Slupik.
p.   cm.   -- (An everything series book)
ISBN 1-58062-741-2
1. Menopause–Popular works. I. Slupik, Ramona. II. Title. III.
Everything series.
RG186 .G46   2003
618.1'75–dc21   2002009827

Many of the designations used by manufacturers and sellers to distinguish their products are claimed as trademarks. Where those designations appear in this book and Adams Media was aware of a trademark claim, the designations have been printed with initial capital letters.

This publication is designed to provide accurate and authoritative information with regard to the subject matter covered. It is sold with the understanding that the publisher is not engaged in rendering legal, accounting, or other professional advice. If legal advice or other expert assistance is required, the services of a competent professional person should be sought.

—From a *Declaration of Principles* jointly adopted by a Committee of the
American Bar Association and a Committee of Publishers and Associations

Illustrations by Barry Littmann.

This book is available at quantity discounts for bulk purchases.
For information, call 1-800-872-5627.

Visit the entire Everything® series at everything.com

Contents

Introduction

CHANCES ARE, IN THE YEARS APPROACHING YOUR OWN MENOPAUSE you have little time for (or interest in) reading up on the subject. You're busy, you're healthy, and you're young! But menopause isn't a condition confined to women who are retired, sick, old, or unfit. Your body won't coordinate its menopause schedule with your appointment book, so you need to know something about the experience in order to be prepared for it. Menopause isn't a horrible condition or dramatic disease—it's an event, a passage, a personal evolution. Your job is to know how you can best care for your body during this time of transition.

So what is menopause? How do you know when you're menopausal? What should you expect from the experience? And finally, what can you do to manage your health through these important years of your life? That's what this book is all about.

There's so much information out there about menopause these days—much of it conflicting or confusing—that it's easy to feel overwhelmed by all of it. And every day new scientific developments change what we know about menopause and the safety and effectiveness of common treatments. In *The Everything® Menopause Book* you find the best of the latest sound, proven information on menopause, presented in simple, no-nonsense terms and an easy-to-use format. This book takes an in-depth look at the symptoms and stages of menopause, options for managing your health through the experience, and important information about hormone replacement therapy and other treatment options. It offers some expert advice for dealing with common symptoms and side effects of menopause, along with important ideas for maintaining a healthy diet and exercise plan to boost your overall physical and emotional fitness during the years preceding, during, and following menopause. You can use this book as a simple, accessible reference of vital information and helpful tips for making the most of your menopausal experience.

And it's also worthwhile to talk a moment about . . . well, talking about menopause. At some point, menopause is a real event in every woman's life—an event that can have important repercussions for anyone who lives with and/or loves a menopausal woman. And although most women won't hesitate to discuss careers, child rearing, and other life issues with friends and family, many women find it difficult to talk about menopause, fearing that it's too personal or socially unacceptable. This book doesn't encourage you to wear a button saying, "Hi, I'm in menopause," and greet every stranger with a handshake and a hearty, "Well, I'm period-free for three months, how about you?" But it does teach some of the many ways that occasional talks with your friends and family about this important experience can be one of the first steps that can make your journey through menopause more meaningful—and less stressful.

Remember, menopause isn't an event defined by a chronological age, and it doesn't mean your life goes "on pause" or grinds to a halt. You can continue to enjoy the same quality of life after menopause that you enjoyed when you were in your forties—maybe even a *better* quality—if you look at the big picture and take some easy, preventative, good-health measures now. The road ahead can be fulfilling and rewarding, especially if you're in the right frame of mind to enjoy it. Keep an open mind, take good care of your body, and explore your options.

CHAPTER 1

Every Woman's Menopause . . . and Yours

As women reach middle age, their world isn't neatly defined by their aging reproductive functions. This chapter helps you explore all of the changes that surround the menopausal experience to help you broaden your perspective of the challenges and opportunities menopause offers.

When Menopause First Gets Your Attention

Menopause doesn't make a grand entrance—no fanfare, no klieg lights, no day and date celebration of a definable event. Menopause becomes a reality for most women through a series of physical, mental, and emotional changes—some subtle, some more dramatic—that tend to emerge, evolve, intensify, and fade over a period of weeks, months, and years. And the changes are unique to each individual, so women don't have a single "menopause profile" to compare themselves to. Menopause can have many faces, and there's no one best way to prepare for or experience it. So how do you know when you are approaching menopause?

Are You Anywhere in This Picture?

Consider the following. You're forty-something and life is pretty good. You've been at your current job long enough to feel that you have things under control (well, sort of). Your ideas and experience have earned you a fair amount of respect in your workplace, and every day you're a little clearer about who you are and where you want to go. Your family is maturing, too; with any luck, you spend less time chauffeuring, cooking, and picking up after others, and more time gardening, working out at the gym, reading, or maybe taking a class at a local community college. Your finances have been improving gradually over the years, and you may have a little more money now to indulge in the things you love best. And you're still young—you look ahead toward many long, happy years of health and well-being.

Of course, everything isn't perfect. Lately, for example, you've been having trouble sleeping—some nights you can't fall asleep, others find you awakening in the middle of the night only to toss and turn your way back to sleep, maybe hours later. When the alarm goes off, you aren't really ready to get up and get going, because you haven't had much real, restorative sleep.

And you suppose the sleep disturbances are to blame for that occasional feeling of tiredness that overtakes you now and again. Some days, in fact, you just feel exhausted—you don't remember that happening much before, do you? And that exhaustion is probably to blame for your memory lapses. Stupid little things, really—sometimes you can't remember why you walked into a room, or what point you intended to make when you began speaking. Thank goodness you're too young to worry about Alzheimer's and senility (aren't you?)!

FACTS

In the year 2000, over 1 million more American women passed the age of forty than in 1999. Every year, the population gets proportionately "greyer"—so don't worry, you have lots of company.

Even so, you find that you don't have much patience with friends and family who want to joke about your forgetfulness, do you? In fact, some days you feel that you could easily snap the head off of the next person that says anything to you. In fact, it sometimes feels like all of your emotions are too close to the surface. Didn't you start crying over a stupid song on the radio when you were driving home last week? That's so unlike you!

But it's probably due to stress; you just need to take more time to relax. One look in the mirror can tell you that you're working yourself too hard, sleeping too little, or not eating and exercising right. Even your skin looks tired, and your hair seems kind of thin and limp. When did that happen?

And not to be too discouraging, but you seem to be putting on a little weight, too, which is totally unfair since you don't eat any more than you used to, and you're working out more. Sure, it's more difficult all the time to resist those cravings for carbohydrates and chocolate, but the weight gain you're experiencing seems way out of proportion to your occasional dietary relapses. What in the heck is going on here?

Is This Perimenopause?

Now, the preceding example may not fit you to a T—you may be in your early forties or even in your late fifties as you approach menopause. You may recognize only a few (maybe even none) of the symptoms listed in the example, while you seem to be experiencing several other symptoms that you don't remember experiencing before. But if any or all of this scenario seems familiar to you, what may be going on is called *perimenopause*—the time preceding menopause (the cessation of all menstrual periods) when associated endocrinological, biological, and clinical changes occur. On average, women begin perimenopause at age forty-seven and experience it for about four years. But women can enter perimenopause in their late thirties or early fifties, and it can last from a few months to eight or ten years. You have no way of knowing precisely when or how you'll begin noticing the changes that announce your coming menopause. Instead, you're more likely to find yourself one day connecting the dots of a number of odd symptoms and changes that eventually add up to the fact that you are, indeed, moving toward menopause.

Whenever it happens, you're likely to have a difficult time accepting the idea that you actually are perimenopausal, but the realization can be a true relief. You may have decided that you were losing your mind or developing an odd and difficult-to-diagnose illness, when in reality, the symptoms you experience are normal, manageable demonstrations of a natural stage in your body's development.

To avoid unnecessary worry and discomfort about menopause, don't deny the obvious. Learn all you can about what's happening to your body, and then take the necessary next steps to begin making your passage to menopause as painless and productive as you possibly can. You've made a great start by picking up this book!

Just the Facts: What Menopause Is and Isn't

According to the Council of Affiliated Menopause Societies (CAMS), menopause is "The permanent cessation of menstruation resulting from the loss of ovarian follicular activity." To put it simply, when you have your last period, you go through menopause. Because your periods may become less regular and occur at greater intervals as you approach menopause, however, you don't know you've gone through menopause until twelve months have passed since your last period. So, by the time you know you've experienced natural menopause, you're already saying, "Been there. Done that" to the whole menopause scene.

Natural versus Induced Menopause

You might have noticed that the preceding sentence mentions "natural menopause." Just as there's no one way to experience menopause, there are multiple types of menopause, too:

- Natural menopause, described previously, is diagnosed when a woman has had twelve months of amenorrhea (no periods) that is not the result of other physical or pathological conditions or treatments.
- Surgical or induced menopause occurs when a woman no longer menstruates as a result of having her ovaries surgically removed (with or without a total hysterectomy) or when ovaries stop functioning, either temporarily or permanently, as a result of chemotherapy, radiation, drug therapy, or other medical treatments.

ESSENTIALS

Note that having a hysterectomy doesn't mean you'll go through menopause. If your uterus is removed but your ovaries remain, your body will continue to produce hormones. In this case, you don't experience menopause as a result of your surgery, even though you won't have monthly menstrual bleeding.

Chemotherapy—the use of drugs to treat cancer—may not result in immediate menopause, but it can damage the ovaries. Depending upon the types of drugs your treatment involves, your ovaries might recover and function normally some time after treatment ends. In some cases, chemotherapy damages ovaries so severely that they cannot produce adequate amounts of hormones. In those cases, menopause may occur months or even years after the therapy has ended. Doctors can't always predict whether damaged ovaries will recover.

Finally, pelvic radiation therapy can cause permanent ovarian failure (and therefore, premature menopause) when the ovaries are the target of high doses of radiation, for example, as treatment for cervical cancer.

Since radiation therapy is a tightly targeted therapy, it often has no effect on ovarian function. If ovaries receive only low doses of radiation, they're likely to fully recover their functions.

Some estimates indicate that one in four women enters an induced or premature menopause. Because the onset of induced menopause is so abrupt, those women have no gradual adjustment period to prepare for postmenopausal changes. Women who have had both ovaries surgically removed, for example, may experience dramatic, abrupt menopausal symptoms, such as severe hot flashes or vaginal dryness.

SSENTIALS   If you face a premature menopause, make sure your doctor discusses all postmenopausal treatment options with you— including hormone replacement therapy.

What Menopause Means

Whatever form of menopause you experience, the results are the same; you stop having periods, you stop being fertile, and you move into the postchildbearing phase of your life. That doesn't mean you become old as a result of menopause; according to the North American Menopause Society (NAM), the average age of natural menopause in the Western world is fifty-one. Most American women born after 1950 can expect to live until their mid-eighties, meaning that the majority of menopausal women in the United States today have one-half to one-third of their lives to live after they've gone through menopause.

But everyone's body is aging all of the time. In menopause, your body undergoes changes that require your attention. Your fluctuating hormones deplete your body's calcium, resulting in bone loss. As you age, you may become more susceptible to heart disease, diabetes, and other illnesses. (Later chapters in this book discuss these changes and how you can best protect yourself from their negative consequences.) Menopause means you need to learn new ways to remain healthy, strong, and vital.

But at the same time, menopause also means that you have an opportunity to enjoy new levels of freedom and self-awareness. You may find that you don't miss the experience of menstruation at all. You no longer have to worry about becoming pregnant, so sex can take on new depths of pleasure. And menopause is a marker of your evolving life; its arrival may encourage you to focus new attention and energy inward, as you take this opportunity to evaluate who you are, what you're doing, and where you want to go next.

What Causes Menopause?

The average woman has about 400 reproductive cycles during her lifetime. In every cycle, the woman's pituitary gland produces follicle stimulating hormones (FSH) that trigger the follicle cells in the ovary that surround the developing eggs to produce estrogen, which in turn prepares an egg (usually just one) for fertilization. As the body's level of estrogen increases, the pituitary gland stops producing FSH and starts producing luteinizing hormone (LH), which causes the ovary to ovulate (release the egg) and produce progesterone, which prepares the uterine lining to accept the fertilized egg.

The mature egg is only one of several "candidates" available each month. Those that don't mature (develop enough to be available for fertilization) are reabsorbed by the body. If the mature egg is unfertilized, it, too, is reabsorbed and the lining of the uterus is shed in the normal menstrual flow. The body's level of estrogen dips, which then triggers the FSH production that starts the whole cycle again.

Every woman is born with a set number of eggs, ranging from 400,000 to 700,000. Half of those eggs deteriorate and are reabsorbed by each girl's body before she reaches puberty. Scientists are still researching why this occurs. With each month's ovulation, more of the egg supply is depleted. As you near menopause, your egg supply diminishes, your follicle cells stop responding to FSH, and you stop ovulating. As a result—over a period of years—you stop menstruating and your ovaries stop making estrogen and progesterone. You may continue to have menstrual periods after you stop ovulating, since your body continues to produce some estrogen. Most women notice a change in the frequency, duration, and flow of their periods during the three to four years before they stop menstruating completely. That's why you can't truly know that you've gone through menopause until a full twelve months have passed since your last period.

SSENTIALS   As the frequency of your ovulation decreases, the FSH levels in your bloodstream increase. In fact, your doctor can test the level of FSH in your blood to determine whether you're nearing menopause, which can be helpful if you're trying to determine your fertility.

What Menopause Means for Your Hormones

Your body produces dozens of hormones, but only three of them play a major role in your reproductive cycle. Those three are estrogen, progesterone, and small quantities of androgens (testosterone, for example). Here's what those hormones do:

- Estrogen is a growth hormone that stimulates the development of adult sex organs during puberty; helps retain calcium in bones; regulates the balance of "good" and "bad" cholesterol in the bloodstream; and aids other body functions, such as blood sugar level, memory functions, and emotional balance.
- Progesterone balances the effects of estrogen by aiding the maturation of body tissues and limiting their growth; stimulates the uterus, breasts, and fallopian tubes to secrete nutrients necessary for the body to prepare for growing an embryo and bearing a child; and raises body temperature and blood sugar levels.
- Androgens are male hormones produced in small quantities by the ovaries and adrenal glands—with the greatest quantities occurring at the midpoint of a woman's cycle—which contribute to a healthy libido by fostering a healthy desire for sex.

Many women incorrectly believe that their bodies stop producing estrogen when they stop ovulating. As your body's supply of egg-producing follicles diminishes, the follicles that remain become less potent and produce lower amounts of estrogen. In perimenopause, cycles become less regular and some ovarian follicles don't mature to ovulation; when that happens, the body's level of progesterone drops.

When the pituitary gland senses that the ovaries aren't producing normal levels of hormones, it produces higher levels of FSH, trying to nudge the ovaries into coughing up more estrogen. And, in the early stages of the perimenopause, that encouragement works; the follicles give up high doses of estrogen, but the body still isn't producing the progesterone that normally rounds out the body's reproductive hormone mix. As a result, a woman in perimenopause may experience widely fluctuating levels of estrogen for a number of years, until the ovaries shut down completely.

When estrogen levels become so low that the lining of the uterus is unable to grow, menstruation stops. The body's FSH levels rise and remain high throughout the postmenopausal years. The body continues to produce small amounts of estrogen, but in levels too small to support the hormone's age-defying functions in the body.

You Aren't the Only Thing That's Changing

Many women today enter their most productive years after the age of forty. Careers are established, children are growing older and more independent, a stronger sense of self emerges, and the pull of pop culture and social trends begin to fade in comparison to a growing inner strength and self-awareness. Although youth and beauty are often considered essential partners, many women are more beautiful at forty than they've ever been before, a result of the increased economic and emotional stability and growing self-confidence that often accompany this period in life.

But most women of forty are also approaching a decade of dramatic personal, physical, and psychosocial change, a new stage of life that may be occurring at a time when they may be uninterested in—and maybe even resistant to—preparing for it. As personal as each woman's perimenopause may be, no woman is alone as she enters this phase of her life.

America Is Maturing

In the United States today, estimates place the number of women over the age of forty at approximately 63 million—over 21.4 million of them are between the ages of forty and fifty. If you're in perimenopause or have experienced menopause, therefore, you're certainly not alone. Most perimenopausal and early postmenopausal women today are part of the Baby Boom generation—and some of them are even Generation Xers (born between 1961 and 1981). These graying generations are among the largest and most influential of the current U.S. population, and they're taking America with them through the menopause experience.

Your Kids Are Maturing

The other women your age around the planet aren't your only companions in incredible change during these years. If you marry and have children in your mid to late twenties or early thirties, by the time you begin experiencing the first signs of perimenopause, it's quite likely that your children may be going through puberty and adolescence.

You went through puberty, so you know what your kids are going through when they hit adolescence. Their bodies and minds are in turmoil. As kids pass through relatively rapid physical changes (some they see as good, others horrify them), they also begin that important first round of "Who am I?" introspection and exploration. They may feel confused, angry, loving, hateful, homely, childlike, adultlike, happy, depressed, bored, excited, and lonely—and that's all just in the first fifteen minutes after they wake up in the morning. If you think the dynamic of an adolescent's raging hormones can wreak havoc on a household, what about combining that loaded pistol with the fluctuating hormonal shifts of a perimenopausal mother?

When you and your child are both trying to figure out who you are and what you want from life, even as you're trying to cope with changing physical and mental patterns in your life, the atmosphere is ripe for conflict. Of course, you also have a rare opportunity to connect with your kid on a whole new level that women who aren't experiencing perimenopause are unlikely to enjoy. But doing so requires a great deal of effort, patience, and creativity on your part. You may or may not be able to turn this dual passage into a positive phase in your family's development, but you do have the opportunity to do so, and it's certainly worth the effort of trying.

Your Mate May Be Menopausal, Too

And what about your life-mate? You don't have to be in a same-sex relationship to experience couples menopause. Though the phenomenon of male menopause was first the subject of research in the 1940s, even twenty years ago you would have had to search for scientific references to male menopause. Today, the medical and psychological communities treat the subject with much more respect.

You've probably heard the worn-out jokes about men going through a midlife crisis—a syndrome that somehow manifests itself in the male's acquisition of a hairpiece, a twenty-something trophy wife, and a shiny red sports car. Well, many men do experience a psychosocial passage known as a midlife crisis, triggered by flagging sexuality, career plateaus, and the realization that having it all isn't all it was cracked up to be. But that midlife event, as important as it may be, isn't the same as male menopause.

Male menopause, known as *andropause* to the medical community, affects (by some reports) nearly 40 percent of men between the ages of forty and sixty. All men begin producing less testosterone after the age of forty. As testosterone levels decrease, men may find that they experience fewer erections, that the erections are less easy to sustain, and that they experience longer intervals between erections. Male menopause can result in a wide range of symptoms in men, including lethargy, depression, mood swings, insomnia, hot flashes, irritability, and decreased sexual desire.

Sexual dysfunction isn't the only marker of male menopause. Studies show that nearly 51 percent of men ages forty to seventy experience some level of impotence in varying degrees of severity and persistence—and that's many more than the number who exhibit symptoms of male menopause.

Diminishing testosterone in the bloodstream isn't the only culprit behind male menopause. Other factors include obesity, excess alcohol consumption, hypertension and the medications used to treat it, lack of exercise, and other "middle-age plagues" that damage health. While medications have been developed to treat erectile dysfunction, testosterone therapy is one of the few nonbehavioral medical treatments available for combating male menopause.

If you are in a same-sex relationship, the chances are very good that at some point you and your mate may both be experiencing symptoms of approaching menopause. Although it may seem that sharing a household with another menopausal woman could lead to increased conflict, you also have a life-partner who may be better able to understand your experience. Both of you will need to remember, however, that every woman's menopause experience is unique, so neither of you can expect the other to have the same symptoms or reactions to those symptoms.

So what does this have to do with your passage through perimenopause and menopause?

If you and your mate are both experiencing the mood swings, irritability, and other negative effects of menopause at the same time, both of you may have a rougher time dealing with the experience. Your partner may or may not understand or accept his or her own struggle with midlife passage, and that could put extra demands on your patience and understanding—at a time when you won't feel particularly well-endowed with either. The essential message here is that your partner may not have the reserves of patience and support necessary to help you through all of the rough patches of menopause, and at times you may have to draw on your deepest supply of those qualities to avoid throwing gasoline on the smoldering fires of family discord.

And What about Your Aging Parents?

And while you're surveying the vast horizon of family change that surrounds you during your perimenopausal years, don't forget about your parents. As you move into your forties, fifties, and sixties, your parents are pushing out ahead of you into the final stages of their lives. They're likely to be dealing with escalating health problems and diminishing self-reliance.

You may find yourself called upon to help your parents make financial decisions, assist with the maintenance of their home, and lend other types of physical and emotional support.

Dealing with elderly parents can be demanding, and you may find these demands hitting you at a time when you're dealing with your own aging process. Facing the realities of aging in your parents can seem especially difficult when you're beginning to feel the effects of age. Expect some stress, and prepare yourself to deal with it.

Don't feel put off if other women in your family didn't (or don't) share your signs and symptoms. Every woman is unique in her perimenopausal experience—even within her own family.

Talking to Friends and Family

As you near fifty, listen to what your friends and contemporaries who aren't experiencing perimenopause say about it (on the rare occasion that the subject comes up). You're likely to hear comments similar to the following.

- "I've made up my mind that I'm just not going to go through all of those symptoms of menopause; I'll fight it to the end!"
- "I don't think it has to be such a dramatic thing; you just have to deal with it."
- "I'll be glad to go through it—I won't miss having periods, believe me."
- "My mom said she didn't even know she was in menopause; her periods just stopped one day, and that was that."

And those comments come from women. Men are more likely to comment on the subject only by making vague references to how much they dread having to deal with a woman in menopause. Then they move on to another topic.

These comments and others like them used to lead anyone to believe that menopause is all a state of mind. You could be strong and simply glide through menopause without giving it the time of day, or you could fall to the sofa in a swoon and whimper for several years, until it was over. This old school of thought tells us that, like a fairy tale monster that feeds on fear, menopause exists only in the imagination and is best defeated by denying its existence. According to this philosophy, you won't have any problems with perimenopause if you simply ignore it. Sounds great, but perimenopause doesn't really work that way.

Communicate to People Who Matter

The information presented in the preceding sections tells quite a different story about what you may expect from perimenopause. Perimenopause and menopause are real medical and psychological events, with some actual indicators and symptoms. Perimenopause is unique to each woman, so no one can know what you're feeling and experiencing during this time. You may experience no symptoms of perimenopause or you may have hot flashes or mood swings that you are certain everyone around you must notice. Bottling up your feelings and trying to hide your perimenopausal symptoms from your family or your close friends may seem like the best thing for them, but in fact, it's unlikely to help anyone—particularly you—understand and deal with the realities of this time in your life.

Though periodic mood swings, anger, and irritability are common in perimenopause, ongoing depression isn't. If your depression lasts more than a few weeks or if your family relationships seem to be on a nonstop downhill slide, talk with your doctor or community mental health service before the problem becomes unbearable.

One of the most important things you can do to make your perimenopausal experience sane and healthy (for you and your friends and family), is to communicate openly with them about your physical and emotional condition. Let your family and friends know what's going on with you. Talk about your symptoms and how they affect your mood, concentration, ability to sleep, level of anxiety, or whatever applies to your experience. Answer their questions and ask for their understanding. If perimenopause is making you irritable and impatient, try to establish some mutual rules for resolving family issues and avoiding unnecessary conflicts. Ask those you care about to help you find a way for everyone to move through the experience and emerge in one piece.

When It's a Family Affair

If you're sharing a life-changing moment with your child, you're going to have to be patient, strong, and attentive. Your spouse or partner may have to step in and take a more active role in parenting, to relieve you of some of the stress and responsibility during certain phases of your perimenopausal changes. You may find that you need a mediator to work through some family difficulties—a relative, counselor, teacher, or family friend.

You and your mate may have to spend more time listening to each other and learning new patterns of behavior. Things are evolving in your life, and therefore, in your relationship. Take this opportunity to revisit the way you think about your lover, life-mate, partner, and friend and to begin interacting with that person on a deeper, more meaningful level.

You can rest assured that your mother and older female relatives have shared at least some portion of your experience in perimenopause. As often as you've felt that you and your mother or other female relatives are from different planets, this is a stop you've all made on your life journey. You may find that this experience offers an opportunity to relate to your family in entirely new ways—and, with any luck, at least some of those ways will be positive!

Give Everyone a Break

Most importantly, try not to waste time judging yourself or your loved ones on the success rate of your communications and relationships during this time. If perimenopause teaches anything, it is that you continue to be a work in progress. Later chapters in this book give you sound advice for making perimenopause an easier, less stressful, and more positive experience. But you can't expect every day to be a golden, glorious success. Every day will offer new challenges and perhaps some new insights and opportunities to learn something new about yourself, your family, your coworkers, and the ways you interact with all of them. If you cut yourself a little slack—accept the fact that once in a while you won't feel and act exactly as you may wish you could—you're more likely to give those around you a little more breathing room, too. Everybody's learning as they go; but when you enter perimenopause, your body signals to you that your life lessons are about to become much more interesting.

CHAPTER 2
Understanding the Symptoms of Perimenopause

Knowing what perimenopause is doesn't really help you understand what it's all about. When you are aware of the range of symptoms women have reported experiencing in perimenopause, you gain a better understanding of the profile of common symptoms and know how to recognize symptoms that masquerade as perimenopause, but may actually point to other issues in your physical and emotional health.

Taking a Closer Look at Perimenopause

As stated in Chapter 1, perimenopause is the period of time preceding menopause in which your body's reproductive system slowly winds down. Though perimenopause differs for every woman it generally marks a time of less-frequent ovulation and fluctuating levels of hormones, including estrogen, progesterone, and FSH. Perimenopause can last anywhere from two to ten years and usually begins sometime in a woman's mid to late forties. Eventually, your ovaries completely stop all egg production and menstruation permanently ceases—that's menopause.

But knowing when and why you stop menstruating doesn't help you prepare to take an active part in managing your health through perimenopause and menopause. In fact, it's rather like being prepared for a trip to France with no more information than your airport names and flight times. Knowing that you fly out of LaGuardia, spend five hours in the air, land at Charles de Gaulle airport, spend ten days in France, then return to LaGuardia from Charles de Gaulle, doesn't do much to help you plan a good trip. And the average statistics of the menopause journey don't tell you much either. Though no one can describe exactly what your experience in perimenopause and menopause will involve, some key bits of information about what others have experienced can help you prepare for the journey.

Consider this chapter your perimenopause orientation session. The goal of the information presented here is to help you feel more comfortable and relaxed when you experience menopause, so you're better able to pass smoothly through every stop along the way, ready and able to deal with any problems you may encounter.

ESSENTIALS

Don't let the term "symptoms" lead you to believe that this chapter is describing perimenopause as a disease or illness—it's neither. Perimenopause is a natural process of physical change. For the sake of simplicity, this book refers to the body's demonstrations of this natural process as "symptoms," with no connotation of illness or disease.

Recognizing the Symptoms

So what can a woman expect from perimenopause? What kinds of symptoms are common—or even possible—and what do they mean? If you have to listen to your body in order to understand its condition and needs, how do you interpret the messages of perimenopausal symptoms? And how do you know if your symptoms are related to perimenopause or some other part of the aging process?

First, it's important to understand that, if you think it may be perimenopause, it probably is. No one is more familiar than you are with your body's feelings and reactions during your monthly cycles. As the following sections demonstrate, women have reported a wide variety of symptoms during and after perimenopause. Remember, some women experience no symptoms at all.

It's also important to keep in mind that everyone can expect to experience some physical and mental signs of aging. As women age, many of their physical changes are triggered or exacerbated by hormonal fluctuations. The good news is, any overt symptom that is associated with changing hormone levels can be temporary—and may even be diminished through diet, exercise, or other therapeutic options. And above all, never forget that everyone's path to menopause takes its own unique course.

What Women Experience in Perimenopause

- "I can't sleep at night; I wake up at two A.M., worried sick about something that won't cause me a moment's concern at two in the afternoon."
- "My periods are spaced further and further apart, but other than that, I haven't had any special symptoms to speak of."
- "Do you think when I wake up in the middle of the night feeling really warm, that could be a sign of something?"
- "First, I'm screaming my head off at my husband, then I feel guilty and depressed about my behavior. Is this the personality I'm going to have for the rest of my life?"

- "I feel like I gain ten pounds every time I look at a donut. I'm trying to exercise more and watch what I eat, but nothing I do seems to slow down my weight gain."

Any of those comments sound at all familiar? Couldn't some of them come from women at any age of their adulthood or couldn't a few of them even have been made by a man?

Perimenopause isn't like measles; you don't wake up one day with a clear sign that you've come down with a case of waning estrogen. So identifying when you enter perimenopause isn't easy. If you start noticing obvious changes in the length of your periods, the intervals between them, or the heaviness of your flow, and you're between the ages of thirty-five and sixty, you should start checking for other signs of perimenopause. But changes in your cycle may not be your first indicator that perimenopause is approaching. Many women report symptoms of perimenopause while their periods remain much the same. Though we all have our own perimenopausal profile, most women feel some or all of the following symptoms as their bodies prepare to stop ovulating:

- Hot flashes
- Mood swings
- Decreased sexual drive
- Weight gain
- Difficulty concentrating
- Heart palpitations
- Migraine headaches
- Irregular and/or heavy periods
- Involuntary urine release and bladder urgency
- Insomnia
- Vaginal dryness and painful intercourse
- Panic attacks

Add to that list everything from aching joints and muscles to the onset of chin whiskers and you've still only started to talk about the wide variety of symptoms perimenopausal women have reported. Though some women report no symptoms of approaching menopause, more women do experience symptoms, so the chances are good that you will, too. Thinning hair, hot flashes, aching joints—these and other symptoms may seem like inevitable side effects of the aging process. But many symptoms of the aging processes can be triggered or exaggerated by the hormonal fluctuations of perimenopause.

Staring Your Symptoms in the Eye

If the preceding list paints an ugly picture of perimenopause, it's also important to mention here that even among women who experience one or more of these symptoms, their effects can be mild, transient, or otherwise unannoying. Your body is adjusting to varying rates of hormones during perimenopause; the signs and symptoms of that adjustment are often temporary, and disappear after your body has acclimated itself to its new hormone levels. The following sections offer you a closer look at the causes of these symptoms so that you have a better idea of what to expect.

FACTS

Don't dismiss symptoms or make up your mind that you're going to tough it out no matter what. You have options for alleviating symptoms—lifestyle changes, behavior modification, hormone replacement therapy, or dietary changes. Do yourself a favor and explore your options.

Hot Flashes (Including Night Sweats!)

Along with irregularities in menses, hot flashes have to earn the dubious honor of being one of the symptoms most commonly reported by women during perimenopause. Nearly 75 percent of women who report perimenopausal symptoms list hot flashes among them. Hot flashes can come at any time of the day or night, but when they occur during sleep, they're usually referred to as night sweats.

Not so long ago many doctors (predominantly men) considered hot flashes to be functions of the female imagination. Today, we know that hot flashes are real, physiological responses to the body's declining levels of estrogen.

Hot flashes can be mild or severe, but in general, they involve a fast-spreading sensation of warmth in your neck, shoulders, and face that may last a few seconds or as long as thirty minutes or more. This sensation may begin at the top of your scalp, behind your ears, on your chest, or even across your nose. Hot flashes don't have to limit themselves to your head and shoulders; many women have also reported flashes occurring across the breasts, below the breasts, or all over the body.

The flashes may be brief and cause only a slight flush on your face, neck, or shoulders; by the time you notice them occurring, they're already beginning to fade. Or, hot flashes can result in dramatic temperature rises that produce profuse perspiration on your upper lip, neck, forehead—or even your entire body. During a severe hot flash, the skin on your face, neck, and scalp may become extremely red, and this flush may take longer to fade than the feeling of "heat" itself. Some women have reported a rapid heart rate immediately before and during their hot flashes; a few women have experienced nausea and/or chills following hot flashes.

ALERT

If you have hot flashes at night, they can contribute to sleeplessness, which can, in turn, contribute to anxiety, tension, mood swings, or even depression. See Chapter 16 for ways to minimize the effects of hot flashes and accompanying night sweats.

Hot flashes may be accompanied by other feelings of physical discomfort, including tension, anxiety, or nervousness. And, if you suffer hot flashes at night, in what most women call night sweats, you may experience some loss of sleep. Many women sleep right through their nighttime hot flashes, and know of them only when they awake in the morning to find their night clothes or pillowcase slightly damp. Severe night sweats can produce such severe heat and sweating that sleep becomes impossible. Extended sleep loss can lead to feelings of anxiety, tension, and even depression. But only a minority of women experiences this severe form of hot flashes.

Irregular and/or Heavy Periods

Even if your periods have always been as regular as clockwork, you can expect some irregularities to occur in the years preceding menopause. As mentioned earlier, as you get older you ovulate less frequently. The levels of estrogen and progesterone produced in your body can flag and surge, contributing to unusually light or skipped periods, or periods that flow for weeks at a time. Some women experience spotting—or even phases of heavy bleeding—for a few days between periods. In other words, you may find that irregularity becomes the norm in your perimenopausal cycles.

What causes cycle irregularity during perimenopause? Once again, the culprit behind the majority of heavy or irregular periods is hormonal fluctuations. In fact, hormone fluctuations can cause a variety of irregularities in your periods. As you enter perimenopause, you might begin to ovulate less frequently. Because all hormone releases are triggered by others, an unusual fluctuation in one hormone can set off a series of unusual fluctuations in others, as your body tries to spur on or hold back the hormone in flux. For that reason, you might have a six-week cycle, followed by a four-week cycle, followed by a six-week cycle with unusually light flow, and so on. (A cycle is the length of time from the first day of one menstrual period to the first day of the next.) Your body is going through a series of starts and stalls as it attempts to adjust to fluctuating levels of hormones in your bloodstream.

Having said that heavy periods and ongoing irregular bleeding are not uncommon during perimenopause, it's also important to have them checked out by your health care provider. Heavy bleeding or bleeding that continues for a long time can be more than an inconvenience. Nonstop heavy bleeding can leave you tired, weak, and anemic—a prime candidate for any cold, flu, or infection you come in contact with. Even more importantly, heavy bleeding may have nothing to do with simple hormonal ebbs and flows. Between 30 percent and 40 percent of all women develop abnormal tissue in the uterus, such as fibroids or polyps, that begin to cause problematic bleeding during perimenopause. Heavy bleeding could also be a sign of precancerous conditions or even endometrial cancer. Don't take chances that your period irregularities are just part of the change. If your irregularities are dramatic, see your health care professional. (For complications of the uterus and their treatment, see Chapter 6.)

If periods come less than twenty-one days apart, last more than a week, are unusually heavy, and maintain these irregularities for more than two cycles, make an appointment with your doctor or health care professional for a gynecological checkup.

Mood Swings

The good news about mood swings is that you may never experience them during perimenopause. But, mood swings are a common complaint of perimenopausal women. Among women who cite symptoms in perimenopause, nearly 50 percent say mood swings are among the symptoms that bother them the most.

Whether you think of them as moodiness, temporary depression, or simply the blues, mood swings can be minor "speed bumps" in your day—or they can leave you feeling totally down and out. The experiences are as individual as the women who have them, but mood swings tend to take the form of intensified emotional reactions. Sometimes, the swing can take you high, and you feel a particularly strong delight in everything around you—the weather, a movie, your dinner companion. Other times, however, mood swings can take you on a wild roller-coaster ride of emotions, such as intense sorrow, despair, love, anger, anxiety, general depression, or fear. A typical anger response during a mood swing can leave your heart pounding, your face flushed, and your head throbbing. Mood swings can trigger bouts of crying and cause deep, dark feelings of hopelessness. Then, as nasty as they can be, mood swings may pass rather quickly, leaving you feeling a bit shaken and confused by the emotional ride.

Though mood swings seem to be emotional responses, they can, in fact, be a direct physical response to the changing hormonal levels in your bloodstream. In fact, many perimenopausal women experience mood swings along with other common symptoms of premenstrual syndrome (PMS), even when those women have never before suffered from PMS symptoms. Those symptoms include a wide range of physical and emotional markers, including gastrointestinal distress, headaches, pains in muscles and joints, fatigue, heart pounding, hot flashes, exaggerated sensitivity to sounds and smells, agitation, and insomnia.

ALERT

Don't confuse mood swings with depression—feelings of despair, hopelessness, lack of energy, and a diluted interest in life around you—with mood swings. When feelings of despair last more than a few weeks, you should consult your doctor. Untreated depression can damage your health and happiness.

Just as mood swings in perimenopause can have both physical and emotional consequences, the causes of those mood swings can be both physical and emotional. First, consider that many of the symptoms of perimenopause can cause emotional distress. Hot flashes can lead to sleeplessness, fatigue, irritability, and anxiety. Those factors alone can make you feel angry, isolated, and under siege—and contribute to occasional moodiness and transient depression.

Involuntary Urine Release

If you've ever experienced urinary tract infections (UTI), you might feel as though they're back with a vengeance during your transition into menopause. And if you've never had urinary tract problems, you might develop them during perimenopause. According to some estimates, nearly 20 percent of all women over the age of forty-five develop some urinary tract problems. Those problems can include UTIs, stress urinary incontinence (caused by a stressor such as sneezing, coughing, or laughing), and urge incontinence (caused by a bladder spasm that forces urine out, even when the bladder is not completely full).

Many women are subject to UTIs on and off throughout their adult lives. But this problem can worsen during perimenopause. Estrogen contributes to the growth and nourishment of all cells and tissues. Because your body produces lower levels of estrogen during the years leading to menopause, the tissues lining the urinary tract can grow thin and more prone to bacterial infection and inflammation. That same lack of estrogen-induced nourishment can weaken the muscles that surround your bladder and urethra. As a result, you experience more UTIs and other urinary tract disorders, a weaker bladder, and less control over urine release.

FACTS

Many urinary tract disorders have similar symptoms, but require different treatments. If you suffer from burning or too frequent urination, involuntary urine release, or a constant full bladder feeling, see your doctor for an accurate diagnosis and treatment.

As mentioned earlier, the most common kinds of urinary tract disorders women experience during perimenopause are stress urinary incontinence, urge incontinence, and UTIs. These disorders can have similar symptoms, but they differ significantly.

Urinary tract infections are caused by bacteria in the urinary tract. The symptoms of UTI include feeling as though you need to urinate all the time, even when your bladder is empty; a burning sensation during urination; and—infrequently—small amounts of blood in your urine. Urinary tract infections can seem to fade, then return again. It's important to remember that, as with any bacterial infections, a full-blown UTI won't go away without antibiotic treatment. If left unchecked, the bacteria that cause a simple bladder infection can spread to the kidneys, causing a much more serious infection called pyelonephritis.

Urge incontinence is the result of a bladder spasm that forces urine out, even when the bladder is not completely full. These involuntary muscle contractions cause the bladder to release urine in varying amounts. Even though the woman may not feel as though her bladder is full and she needs to urinate, the sight, sound, or even thought of water or urination can cause the sudden reflex need to urinate and an accompanying release of urine.

Stress urinary incontinence is another cause of periodic involuntary urine release. But unlike urge incontinence that can result from the mere thought of emptying the bladder, stress incontinence usually has a specific triggering event, such as a sneeze or cough. Some women release small amounts of urine when they bend over, laugh, or exercise.

Stress urinary incontinence is caused by weakened sphincter muscles, which surround the urethra, and can occur in women of any age. Women who have given birth, especially very large babies or difficult vaginal deliveries, often experience this disorder many years before they approach menopause. But during menopause, weakening sphincter muscles can contribute to the onset of stress urinary incontinence, even in women who have never experienced it. Obesity and chronic lung conditions that produce a lot of coughing, such as emphysema or cigarette smoking, can also cause or aggravate the condition. Certain strengthening exercises called the Kegel exercise, postmenopausal hormone therapy, and even surgery are just some of the treatments used to combat this disorder. Losing weight and quitting smoking help, too.

FACTS

A number of therapies can help end many urinary tract disorders. Biofeedback, pelvic floor muscle exercises (known as Kegel exercise), and medication are just some treatment possibilities. Weight loss and bladder retraining can be successful tools in fighting incontinence, too. Talk with your doctor to learn more.

Changes in Libido

Few things are more individual than libido. Everyone has a unique attitude toward sex and sexuality, and certainly, we all differ in our sexual habits and desires. While this undeniable (and delightful!) individuality may seem to contradict any generalizations about how sexual desire can change during menopause, many women do experience some types of changes during this time.

Many studies—including those of the famous Alfred Kinsey—indicate that both men and women can experience gradually declining sexual desire as they age. Pay special attention to the "can" in that last sentence. It's important to remember that not everyone undergoes any noticeable change in libido during menopause—in fact, many women don't. Still, many women in perimenopause have reported noticeable changes in their level of sexual desire. Some say they have more interest in sex and enjoy it more, while others say their desires have diminished, and still others say they find sex increasingly unappealing—even painful. If menopause is the trigger for this change, how can it differ so radically from one woman to another?

To understand the answer to that question, remember that human sexuality is a complex and somewhat mysterious force, and changes in sexual desire are rarely explained by simple answers or attributed to single sources—no matter when those changes occur.

ESSENTIALS

It's also important to remember that every woman's unique mind, body, relationships, attitudes, and environment help shape her sexual response. Her self-image and level of self-confidence play a supreme role. Understanding some of the physical and emotional factors that can impact libido during perimenopause and menopause is an important first step in understanding your own sexual experience during this time of transition.

Hormones play a critical role in your body's sexual response. Estrogen increases blood flow to all of your body's tissues, and it helps keep the walls of your vagina well-nourished and healthy. Estrogen also helps maintain normal vaginal secretions and contributes to vaginal moistness and flexibility. As your body's hormone levels fluctuate through perimenopause and then diminish after menopause, you might experience some concurrent decline in sexual desire.

But that's not the whole story. Let's not forget those many women who report that their sex lives improve at this stage of life. The reasons for this not unusual phenomenon are relatively easy to understand. As women move into perimenopause and menopause, they may have more access to quality time with a sexual partner. As children become more independent and then leave the family, interruptions and distractions diminish, allowing sex to be unhurried and spontaneous. After menopause, women can stop worrying about birth control, and therefore enjoy lovemaking free from unwanted pregnancy. And the growing self-confidence that comes with maturity can be a real turn-on—to both the woman and her partner.

Weight Gain

The results are in; weight gain is commonly seen as people of both sexes age. And that isn't exactly new information. The term "middle age spread" was coined decades ago to describe the tendency of the postforty body to take on excess weight. Now everyone doesn't gain weight during perimenopause and after menopause, and not everyone who does gain weight gains debilitating amounts. But, the fact is that the majority of women report weight gain at this time. Even women who don't gain weight may experience a change in their body shape. Many women in middle age gain softer, rounder abdomens, larger hips, thicker waistlines, and even extra weight on their shoulders, arms, and thighs.

Your body's metabolism changes as you move into middle age. As you age, your body burns calories much more slowly (some studies say by as much as 4 to 5 percent) as each decade passes. So, instead of burning off the calories that you eat, your body converts them into fat. You may feel as though you aren't eating any more, and may actually feel you are eating less, but your body's furnace just needs less fuel to perform the same functions.

Although you may feel as though you are always on your feet and very active, many people slow down a bit as they move into middle age— running fewer errands, doing less physical work around the house, and so on. All of these factors contribute to unwanted—and sometimes unhealthy—weight gain during perimenopause and after menopause.

Difficulty Concentrating

If you're approaching fifty, and it seems as though you aren't quite as sharp mentally as you used to be, it's probably because you aren't. Though fuzzy thinking, forgetfulness, difficulty concentrating, and memory problems are common complaints of perimenopausal and menopausal women, these issues are linked as closely with the aging process as they are to changing ovarian functions. Today, doctors and health care professionals recognize that certain cognitive problems are due to depleted estrogen levels and other changes in the aging brain.

QUESTIONS?

Can estrogen supplements help women in perimenopause think more clearly?
Some of the brain's midlife slowdown results from loss of healthy neurons. Some studies have shown that estrogen can help heal damaged neurons and increase other neurotransmitters that govern memory and other mental functions, but other studies haven't supported these results. Studies continue, so watch for developments.

How does this fuzzy thinking manifest itself? In ways you've probably experienced most of your life, for example, losing your car keys, forgetting what you were about to say, recognizing a face but failing to recall the name, searching fruitlessly for the right word, being easily distracted, or losing your train of thought. As women reach the age of menopause (around age fifty), however, they can suffer an increase in these sorts of problems. You may have heard people refer to these lapses as "senior moments," and if you're approaching the age of menopause you're likely to be experiencing them, yourself. The aging process affects the brain, as it does in all the other parts of the body.

While you can't stop your brain's odometer from registering the passing years, you can slow down and repair many of the issues that contribute to fuzzy thinking and other cognitive roadblocks. See Chapter 19 for more information.

Heart Palpitations

Heart palpitations are the sudden uncomfortable awareness that your heart is pounding, often at a more rapid rate than normal. Heart palpitations can be frightening, but remember that they aren't uncommon in perimenopausal and menopausal women. Certainly these women aren't the only ones to experience palpitations—many men and women have them after exercising, when frightened, or while taking some medications. But at menopause, the instances of heart palpitations seem to rise in women. Their frequency and severity vary from woman to woman, but under normal circumstances they aren't a problem. If they get out of hand, however, occurring in rapid succession, heart palpitations can cause problems.

Women describe heart palpitations differently, but in general a heart palpitation feels like your heart is beating rapidly, out of sequence, too strenuously, or in some other abnormal fashion. A heart palpitation can feel like no more than a brief fluttering in your chest that passes within a matter of a few seconds. Other, stronger palpitations can feel like a distinct pounding in your chest that lasts a few minutes and can leave you feeling light-headed or short of breath.

If your heart palpitations are severe or produce significant discomfort or side effects, you need to talk to your doctor or health care provider about them. Some palpitations are a warning sign of an impending heart attack. Pay attention to the number and frequency of your palpitations, and be pre-pared to discuss these and your heart history when you talk with your doctor.

Heart palpitations can be caused by anxiety or some other system-stimulating problem, such as too much caffeine or an overactive thyroid gland. Blood sugar levels that are either too high or too low can also contribute to heart palpitations. Palpitations that are present upon awakening are particularly worrisome. As you move into perimenopause, your body's fluctuating hormone levels can contribute to all of these causes. The good news about this symptom is that heart palpitations associated with perimenopause and menopause tend to run their course and stop after the body adjusts to postmenopausal hormone levels.

Caffeine, cigarettes, and excess sugar can oversimulate your system and be a contributing factor in heart palpitations. Perimenopause is a great time to cut back on your intake of these.

Migraine and Other Headaches

Technically, migraine headaches aren't considered a symptom of menopause. Nevertheless, many women who have never experienced a migraine in their lives begin having them during perimenopause. These hormonally related migraines are often experienced by younger women in the few days before their periods. In both cases, fluctuations in your body's estrogen levels seem to be a cause.

Though both sexes suffer from migraines, women are three times more likely to have them. Migraines are intensely painful headaches thought to be associated with constricted blood vessels in the brain. Women who suffer migraines describe them as pounding headaches that can cause nausea, vomiting, and a strong sensitivity to light, noise, and odors. Some migraine sufferers—almost one-third, according to some studies—report a certain premonition, or aura, for several minutes before the actual pain begins. This aura can include flashing lights, certain odors, changes in their vision, or numbness in a hand, arm, or leg. Migraines usually last four or more hours, and they can last as long as a week.

Migraines aren't the only kind of headaches that seem to accompany perimenopause. In general, women report having more frequent and severe headaches during this time. These are usually simple stress or muscle tension headaches, and are often relieved by over-the-counter analgesics such as aspirin and acetaminophen.

Insomnia

Interruptions in normal sleep patterns are common complaints of perimenopausal and postmenopausal women. During the years approaching menopause, many women find that they wake once or twice during the night and then have a difficult time returning to sleep. Other times, women find that it takes longer for them to fall asleep when they go to bed at night or that they awaken an hour or two earlier than they used to. Whatever form it takes, insomnia leaves women feeling tired, irritable, and out of touch with their surroundings.

This chapter has already discussed many other conditions of perimenopause that logically contribute to sleeplessness—night sweats, anxiety, and the need for frequent urination. But the root causes of insomnia during these transitional years go even deeper. As we age, most people establish new sleep patterns. Although some women go through a phase during perimenopause in which they actually require much more sleep than they have previously, others experience periods of wakefulness and restlessness during hours that they previously would have been deeply asleep. Stress, changes in diet, the need for frequent urination, heartburn, hot flashes, and anxiety are a few of the different factors that can trigger insomnia. And, the factors that prevent you from falling asleep when you first go to bed at night can be very different from those that wake you and keep you awake in the middle of the night.

Most health care professionals agree that certain lifestyle habits can contribute to insomnia—at any time in your life. Get regular exercise and try not to consume any alcohol, sugar, caffeine, or rich foods within the two to three hours before bedtime.

Fortunately, many women find that insomnia is a transient problem that may last no more than a few months. For others, insomnia during perimenopause may be so severe that it hampers their performance and sense of well-being during the day. Chapter 10, "Your Mind, Mood, and Emotional Health," offers a number of good options for minimizing insomnia when it strikes. As always, if your symptoms become severe, consult your doctor or health care professional. You can combat insomnia, so don't allow it to drag you down during this important transition phase.

Stay on Top of Your Symptoms

As you have seen in this chapter, a wide range of symptoms can appear during the years preceding menopause. But it's important to remember that, as noted at the beginning of this chapter, you may experience none, some, or all of these symptoms—or others that aren't even listed. To be certain that you are doing all you can to maintain peak health during this important time of transition, pay close attention to your body, and don't ignore the messages it sends you. Many of the symptoms that initially seem par for the course for middle age, may be symptoms of problems requiring serious and quick medical treatment. So don't ignore any ongoing problem because you think it's just the change. Work closely with your health care provider to make sure that your body gets any and all of the help that it needs to stay strong, fit, and healthy.

CHAPTER 3

Passing Through
the Stages

Since women of fifty today may have more than one-third of their lives ahead of them, it's important that they understand the changes their bodies are experiencing. Tracking the progress of your own journey toward and through menopause will help you feel more comfortable and secure about where you are—and ready to enjoy the years ahead.

A Traveler's Guide to Menopause

When we talk about the stages of perimenopause and menopause, we're really talking about the normal aging process—a subject that's become nearly taboo in our youth-oriented Western culture. Fortunately for America's burgeoning postfifty population, however, aging today is a happier, healthier business than it was even thirty years ago. We're living longer, healthier lives now. Medical advancements have made the age of fifty more of a midway marker than the opening of the final scene that it used to be. Remember, menopause isn't really something you go through, although that's often the easiest way to describe the period of change most women experience in the years preceding and following full, natural menopause. Menopause is merely one event in the long journey women make as they move away from their reproductive years and into their postreproductive years.

This transformation takes place in stages that occur, for most women, over a period of decades. Although every woman's body chemistry and, therefore, age experience is unique, many experts agree that most women typically experience the following physical changes on the menopause journey, however.

- **Perimenopause**—the years when a woman's estrogen production gradually decreases as a natural result of aging—typically occurs during a woman's midforties.
- **Menopause**—the time when ovulation ceases and estrogen production falls to such low levels that all menstruation stops for at least twelve months in the case of natural menopause or immediately in the case of surgical or induced menopause. Many women enter natural menopause in their fifties.
- **Postmenopause**—the years following menopause.

The following sections detail each of these stages. But, to put the changes that occur in perimenopause in perspective, take a moment to review the starting point from which most women embark on the journey toward menopause.

The term premenopause is no longer used to refer to the years preceding menopause, because all the years of a woman's life that precede menopause are premenopause. Today, perimenopause is used to describe the years when a woman's reproductive system slows down as it approaches menopause.

The Phases of Menstruation

Women in their teens, twenties, and early thirties who have typical reproductive functions experience monthly menstrual cycles. Some people label these years as "the reproductive years," but it's important to remember that as long as you ovulate and have periods, you are fertile and you can conceive. For the purposes of this book, therefore, just think of this life stage as that of your early adulthood, which lasts, for the average woman, into her forties.

By the time most women reach their late teens, they ovulate regularly, and their bodies establish their "normal" reproductive cycle. Although the length and regularity of the cycle varies from woman to woman, you can think of the typical reproductive cycle as occurring in two main phases:

- **Buildup—(follicular phase),** the time when one of the ovaries begins developing an egg for release, starting on the first day of menstrual bleeding and continuing until midway through the cycle when ovulation occurs.
- **Premenstrual—(secretory phase),** the time following ovulation when the uterine lining develops in preparation for nourishing a potential fertilized egg.

Hormones trigger each event that occurs during the two phases of one complete menstrual cycle. Here's a rough overview of what happens:

1. On Day 1 of the menstrual cycle, the body begins to shed its built-up uterine lining and the pituitary gland releases follicle stimulating hormones (FSH) to prompt the ovaries to produce estrogen in order

to prepare an egg for ovulation, which develops in one follicle in one ovary. (Occasionally more than one egg matures in the same cycle.)

2. FSH levels pulse occasionally through the next thirteen days as estrogen levels gently rise to their peak.

3. Around Day 14 the pituitary gland releases luteinizing hormone (LH) to make the ovary release the egg and to turn the follicle cells that surrounded the egg into a progesterone-producing machine.

4. For the next two weeks or so, estrogen production slowly diminishes as progesterone production steps up, and the two hormones work together to spur the lining of the uterus to thicken in preparation for accepting and nourishing the fertilized egg.

5. Toward the end of the cycle (around Day 28), the egg reaches the uterus. If fertilized, the egg embeds in the lining and estrogen and progesterone levels remain strong. If the egg is unfertilized, all hormones—FSH, LH, estrogen, and progesterone—drop to minimum levels and the lining of the uterus begins to fall away as menstrual flow, which takes us back to Day 1 of the cycle.

ESSENTIALS

According to some studies, your menstrual cycles may shorten before age forty, then lengthen slightly as you approach menopause. So, while your period may occur every twenty-six days when you're forty years old, as you reach forty-five, thirty-five-day cycles may be normal for you.

This cycle may take twenty-one days in some women, or as many as thirty-five days in others. Studies have shown that your age may play a critical role in the length of your menstrual cycle. If your cycles fall outside this range, you should discuss it with your doctor.

Fast Facts about Premenstrual Syndrome

Even when you've established your own individual cycle and are in the height of your reproductive years—from your late twenties through midthirties—your monthly cycle may not proceed as a smooth ride. Most women experience some symptoms associated with their menstrual periods, including cramps, swollen and tender breasts, mood shifts, and headaches. These symptoms can also be present—along with others—in premenstrual syndrome (PMS). Some research indicates that PMS can include as many as 150 separate systems, but all symptoms of PMS fall into two major categories:

- Physical symptoms of PMS include bloating, water retention, pelvic pressure or cramping, and headaches or migraines.
- Emotional symptoms can consist of irritability, mood swings, difficulty concentrating, and food cravings.

Some women never have PMS, while others—some studies estimate one-third of all women—may have episodes of it throughout their adult lives. These women often find that PMS is most frequent and severe during their thirties. Many women who have never experienced PMS or have had only occasional, minor symptoms, report severe PMS phases as they enter perimenopause.

Although PMS symptoms can occur anywhere from midway through your cycle to a few days after you begin your period, no one symptom should ever last more than two weeks. If you have any symptom longer than fourteen days, report it to your doctor.

A less common but even more debilitating type of premenstrual syndrome is premenstrual dysphoric disorder (PMDD). Women who suffer from PMDD often experience severe depression, anxiety, sleep disturbances, and fatigue in addition to a wide range of physical disturbances. Though these two syndromes differ in severity, diagnosis, and treatment, both seem to be linked to the way the body processes and responds to reproductive hormones. (See Chapter 11 for more information.)

Doctors diagnose PMS and PMDD based on when a woman's symptoms occur, not just the symptoms themselves. If you want to track your own premenstrual symptoms, you can keep a menstrual journal. If symptoms repeat at specific intervals, they may indicate PMS.

The Journey Through Perimenopause

During perimenopause you may experience the classic symptoms discussed in Chapter 2, including irregular and/or heavy periods, mood swings, hot flashes, weight gain, and headaches.

Or you may experience increased severity of PMS symptoms. PMS and some symptoms of perimenopause mirror each other because both are thought to be caused by fluctuating levels of reproductive hormones. Some women are more sensitive to these fluctuations than others, which explains why some women have no symptoms and others have symptoms that are severe.

SSENTIALS

Don't read too much into new and more severe PMS symptoms. Although they can signal that your reproductive system is slowing down—and that means that you're moving into perimenopause—they can also signal a new awareness of your body, or your body's reaction to life's increasing stresses.

Chronicle Your Symptoms

But how do you know whether or not you're truly experiencing perimenopause? Your doctor or health care professional can help determine that with tests discussed later in this chapter. But remember—most diagnoses of perimenopause aren't based on symptoms so much as on when symptoms occur. So if you have begun to notice changes in your monthly cycle or other symptoms associated with perimenopause, you can begin the diagnostic process yourself by keeping a menstrual calendar.

You can use any system that works for you, but here's an example of how the menopause calendar can work. Perhaps you have been experiencing periodic waves of anxiety and depression, along with bad headaches and occasional hot flashes. And occasionally your craving for sweets and carbohydrates gets totally out of control. You can use a menopause calendar to track those symptoms, to see if they're associated with specific days of your monthly cycle.

To begin, you need a simple calendar—you can use a desktop calendar, appointment book, wall calendar, electronic calendar file, a journal, or any medium you choose, as long as your calendar lists days and dates and provides room for you to record your daily notes. To save room, devise some abbreviations for symptoms and events, such as:

H	Headache
An	Feeling Anxious
CC/SC	Carbohydrate Cravings/Sweet Cravings
D	Depressed
HF	Hot Flash
P	Period (Menstrual)
GM	General Mood

Finally, you need to have a rating system to rank the severity of your symptoms. That way, if you have a mild headache one day and a migraine another, you can track the difference. Similarly, you can note how light or heavy your flow was on any day of your period. You may choose to rank severity with a scale of 1 to 5, with 1 being least severe/lightest and 5 being most severe/heaviest. You can use this ranking to note your general mood, too, with 5 meaning "feeling horrible" and a 1 indicating that you're feeling great. Add new symptoms as they occur, so you can get a full picture of how your health and how you feel changes from day to day. Don't be compulsive about your calendar, but make sure it notes cyclical symptoms and menopause dates. Some doctors or health care providers might even offer you their own standard version of a symptom calendar, like the one shown in **FIGURE 3-1**.

FIGURE 3-1: MENSTRUAL SYMPTOM DIARY

You can begin tracking your symptoms on any day you choose, though some like to start on the first day of their period. Here's one example of a menstrual symptom calendar.

Name:

Weight (cycle day 1):

Severity of symptoms:

None   Moderate

Mild   Severe

Cycle Day	1	2	3	4	5	6	7	8	9	10	11	12	13	14	15	16	17	18	19	20	21	22	23	24	25	26	27	28	29	30	31	32	33	34	35
Date																																			
Menses																																			
Nervous tension																																			
Mood swings																																			
Irritability																																			
Anxiety																																			
Depression																																			
Forgetfulness																																			
Crying																																			
Confusion																																			
Insomnia																																			
Weight change*																																			
Swelling of extremities																																			
Breast tenderness																																			
Abdominal bloating																																			
Headache																																			
Craving for sweets																																			
Increased appetite																																			
Heart pounding																																			
Fatigue																																			
Dizziness or faintness																																			

*Please record the difference between today's weight and the weight on cycle day one. For example, if you weighed 140 on the first day of your period and now you weigh 143, enter +3; or if you weigh 145, enter +5.

Every day, note on your calendar any symptoms you experience and their severity ranking. Note the first and last days of your period, and how light or heavy your bleeding is each day. Keep the calendar for at least three months to get a good roadmap of recurring symptoms and your cycle's regularity or irregularity. This information can help you—and your health care provider—spot symptoms that might be associated with perimenopause.

Many women have found that simply tracking and understanding the cyclical nature of their perimenopausal symptoms make those symptoms less severe and intrusive. For example, if on the twenty-first day of your cycle every month you're prone to feeling anxious or depressed, but that the feeling passes by Day 23, those feelings may seem less severe and debilitating. If you expect to develop a sore throat sometime within the second week of your cycle, you aren't worried by its appearance every month. Don't misunderstand this message—keeping a menstrual calendar won't cure your perimenopause symptoms. But information is power; the more you know, the better able you are to make strong, informed decisions about how to respond to your symptoms.

If you have a sudden onset of extreme symptoms—such as severe headaches or extremely heavy bleeding—that lasts more than a few days, see your health care provider. Severe long-lasting symptoms may be related to some serious illness or disease. You need to report them right away.

If You Need to Talk to Your Doctor

When your symptoms of perimenopause cause too much disruption in your life, it's time to talk to your doctor. Health care providers can help to determine whether or not perimenopause and its accompanying hormonal shifts are contributing to the symptoms you're experiencing, and how you best can treat them. Doctors can test for conditions of perimenopause by checking hormone levels in your blood. (Newer saliva tests are currently being developed, but most medical experts don't yet consider them reliable.) Those tests may check for levels of estrogen, FSH, and LH—your doctor determines which hormones to check, based on your symptoms and health history. Rising levels of FSH, for example, can indicate that the body is ovulating less frequently, and therefore FSH is being released from the pituitary gland in greater quantities to help spur on the ovaries' production of estrogen. Many health care providers consider an FSH level of forty or above to be a firm indicator that menopause has occurred. FSH levels can fluctuate in perimenopause, so sometimes a single test doesn't provide enough information on which to base a diagnosis.

ESSENTIALS

The point of keeping your menstrual and PMS symptom calendar is to show it to your doctor, so remember to take it with you to your appointment. Some hormone testing may be best performed on certain days, and your doctor will need the information you've tracked to determine when to schedule your test.

If your doctor diagnoses you as being perimenopausal, he or she will talk to you about possible treatment options. Chapter 11, "Understanding Hormones and HRT," and Chapter 12, "Alternatives to Hormone Replacement Therapy," will give you more information on these topics. Remember, your symptoms may go through a number of changes or even resolve themselves with no treatment at all. In fact, some estimates say that as many as 55 percent of women in perimenopause use no treatment of any kind. In many cases, your body slowly adjusts to its changing hormone levels, and your symptoms remain mild or even unnoticeable. (Unfortunately, most women whose menopause is artificially induced have more pronounced, severe symptoms, and are more apt to require hormone replacement therapy or other treatment options.)

If you're in perimenopause, you have a number of options, and your health care provider can help you explore all of them. It's important that you have a doctor that you feel completely comfortable with at this important time. Chapter 5, "Working with Your Doctor," discusses that relationship.

Other Physical Changes During Perimenopause

Recognizing the unique experience each of us has as we age, most of us can expect to experience other physical changes during—and perhaps as a result of—the physical changes of perimenopause. If perimenopause occurs during a woman's forties, for example, here are some of the changes her body might be undergoing:

- Muscles may lose mass easier and become harder to tone during your forties, so your old workout plan may not be enough to maintain the strength and body weight you enjoyed in your thirties. You may need a new workout program during this time; see Chapter 14.
- Bones can start to lose calcium as estrogen levels recede and the body becomes less efficient at absorbing calcium from food. You may need to adjust your diet to include more vitamin D and calcium, or consider taking supplements. See Chapter 8 for more information.
- Eyes become less efficient as the lenses lose elasticity and their controlling muscles weaken, making focusing close-up more difficult. Estrogen helps keep eyes and muscles elastic, so diminishing levels of estrogen contribute to this degeneration.
- Skin and hair can begin to thin in response to lowered levels of estrogen; most people start to get some grey hair in their forties. Estrogen also helps maintain the collagen content (the basic protein bridgework) of your skin, thus keeping it youthful and elastic. Your strong ally in the battle against this aging factor is a healthy diet and lots and lots of water. See Chapter 15 for more information.
- Metabolism slows down during your forties, so weight gain can creep up on you, even if you maintain your previous diet and workout plan. Typical dieting methods are unlikely to work as well for you at this age, so maintaining or losing weight may require additional exercise and calorie cutting.
- Propensities for certain conditions such as diabetes and asthma can accelerate during this time, due to changing hormone levels, lowered resistance to stress and infections, and other factors of aging. Medical checkups and health maintenance are more essential than ever at this point; see Chapter 6.

Don't be put off by this list; yes, the aging process does involve physical changes and even some deterioration of your body's systems.

But there's never been a time when medicine and health care, public information, and healthy life practices have been better able to contribute to everyone's pursuit of a healthy, active middle age. You have more control than any generation that's preceded you in how quickly or slowly your body loses ground to the aging process. You can learn ways to manage the effects of perimenopause and its role in the aging process.

If you've been casual about your health until you hit forty (which most of us are), now is a perfect time to get serious about preparing for a long, healthy life ahead. Diet, exercise, lifestyle changes, and regular medical checkups are your strongest agents for maintaining a strong, healthy body.

Menopause and the Years Ahead

If you still have both of your ovaries as you move into your fifties, the chances are good that you'll stop having menstrual periods altogether. When you've not had a period for twelve months, it's official—you've experienced natural menopause. So you stop having periods—but what other changes take place as a result of this transition? And what lies ahead?

Hormones Take a Dive after Menopause

After menopause, estrogen and progesterone levels plummet. Although other parts of your body continue to produce some hormones, they cannot compensate fully for the loss of ovarian hormone production. The specific role of these hormones is treated in Chapter 11, but some of the major postmenopausal side effects are increased bone loss and the drying and shrinking of the vagina (vaginal atrophy). Fewer vaginal secretions are produced when there is no estrogen, so your vaginal wall becomes less lubricated and flexible and more prone to tears and cracking. In fact, all of your skin tissue becomes thinner and less elastic, including the muscles that surround your urethra (the opening to the bladder). That's how diminishing hormone levels can contribute to involuntary urine release through stress incontinence.

Your cardiovascular system misses those hormones, too, with their beneficial impact on HDL cholesterol and their inhibiting effect on LDL cholesterol. And just as your arteries become more susceptible to plaque buildup, they begin to narrow and lose elasticity. As a result, estrogen loss can contribute to heart disease.

Another important side effect of plummeting hormones is a rapid advance of the bone loss that began in your forties. In the first five years that follow menopause, women can lose as much as one-fourth of their bone density—a potentially deadly development. Bone fractures that develop as a result of osteoporosis can have life-threatening consequences. This bone loss slows down for most women within a decade or so of menopause, but without supplements or HRT, it continues throughout a woman's life.

FACTS

Hot flashes can continue for a period of years after menopause, but in most cases, diminish entirely within five years. See Chapter 16, "Coping with Hot Flashes," for ways to minimize the burn of hot flashes.

Other Postmenopausal Changes

During your fifties and early sixties—the decades immediately following menopause—your body undergoes some inevitable changes resulting from the natural aging process. Again, your body is unique, and so are your family medical history, your lifestyle, and your individual health program. But in general, here are the types of changes many women experience in the years that follow menopause:

- Hearing loss can set in, due to the ear canal tissue's becoming thinner and drier. Many people have no hearing loss until they are in their sixties, but almost one-third of women over sixty-five report hearing problems. Keep this loss to a minimum by protecting your ears from loud noises. Wear earplugs when you mow the lawn and avoid sitting close to loud stereos and televisions. And get annual hearing checkups, so you know when your hearing loss reaches the you-need-a-hearing-aid stage.

- Joints lose cartilage with age and connective tissue becomes less flexible and resilient, making arthritis and other types of joint pain more common in aging women. Exercise and weight control are critical factors in maintaining healthy joints.
- Lungs become less elastic as we hit our midfifties, which can contribute to shallower breathing and, therefore, less oxygen in our bloodstream. Get plenty of aerobic exercise to keep your lungs pumping. And, if you're still smoking, quit now!
- The brain loses mass and shrinks slightly with each passing year. As a result, women can face impaired cognitive functions as early as age seventy. Keep your body and mind active—participate in a regular aerobic exercise program, work crossword puzzles, learn to use the computer, visit with family and friends, read the newspaper, and travel. Life's pleasures are also your best weapon in keeping your mind alert and agile. Remember, if you use it, you don't lose it.
- Digestion slows down as we reach our sixties, and food moves at a slower pace through our intestines. As a result, many postmenopausal women report problems with constipation. Eat plenty of whole grains, fresh fruit, and vegetables, and drink plenty of water to combat this change in your digestive function (and, you guessed it, exercise).

Living for the Rest of Your Life

These changes contribute to the challenges you face in maintaining your strength and health as you move through the postmenopausal years of your life. Though aging is inevitable, you exercise tremendous control over its effects. Menopause demands that you pay attention to your body, make decisions, and take actions that can protect and nurture it throughout the many years ahead. But menopause also can usher in a time of great freedom, personal exploration, and growth. How you manage the symptoms of perimenopause and the realities of aging that follow will determine your own postmenopausal experience. The remaining chapters of this book take a closer look at all the health issues that surround menopause, and offer simple, effective, smart ideas for managing your health and combating these issues—now and for the rest of your life.

CHAPTER 4

Why Your Attitude Matters

As you approach menopause, you may not have evaluated your attitude toward the transition you are making. The way you think about menopause, aging, change, and your own self-worth is all-important at this time of physical and emotional transition. This chapter offers you some key techniques for assessing just how you feel about menopause—what hopes and fears you bring with you to perimenopause and menopause.

Is It Time to Check Your Attitude?

Women approaching menopause today have much to be thankful for. At no previous time in history have we known more about both the biology and psychology of menopause and aging. We've never had more therapeutic options for taming the symptoms of menopause. We have an unprecedented understanding of diet and nutrition and the role they play in healthy aging. Women, though still struggling for equality in many areas, have trampled down many of the old barriers of sexual stereotypes and discrimination. Many women in their fifties are just entering the best years of their professional careers. Attitudes toward women and their roles and worth in society are changing, as are attitudes toward the experience of menopause and those women who are in it.

But this may be a good time to rethink some of your most deep-rooted ideas. This chapter acknowledges and evaluates some of the "truths" you've learned about menopause and aging over the years, and how those ideas can affect your attitude toward your own experience. It also takes a closer look at some of the myths and fears that surround menopause, even in today's enlightened social climate, and offers some simple techniques for tracking unproductive and unhealthy beliefs to their source and cleaning them out of your mental closet. Menopause is a positive experience, and the final sections of this chapter focus on the real benefits you gain as you pass into this phase of your life. It's easy for you to believe the worst about menopause; now, it's time to see menopause for what it is—and what it can be.

This Isn't Your Mother's Menopause

If you're fifty years old today—one year younger than the average age of menopause in the United States—you were born sometime around 1951, and (on average), your mother was born between the years of 1920 to 1932. She probably went through menopause sometime in the 1970s or early 1980s. Think about those dates for just a moment and consider how much society has changed during that time. When your mother was born, little was said about menopause and few women would have felt comfortable talking about "the change" even within a group of friends. Today, it's not unusual for menopause to be the subject of happy hour chatter. So, much of what we say about menopause has changed—but how about the way we think about menopause? Has our basic set of ideas and beliefs about menopause gone through a true evolution?

What Our Mothers Taught Us

By the time your mother went through menopause, the first 1976 International Conference on Menopause was under way, and television's Edith Bunker had brought the *M* word to prime time, when her transition into menopause became the subject of a series of episodes of the popular "All in the Family" television sitcom. Nevertheless, the 1970s and 1980s weren't years of great advancements in the public's understanding of menopause.

If you ask many women in their fifties today what their mothers told them about menopause, they're likely to respond, "She never mentioned it to me." If society was breaking down the barriers that deemed menopause an unacceptable topic, why wasn't more information available about menopause during the 1970s and 1980s? Much of the lack of new information about menopause during this time was the result of a shortage of good menopause research prior to the last quarter of the twentieth century. And, the research that was being conducted wasn't available to the general public; these were pre-Internet years, remember, and newspapers and television shows weren't likely to report new findings in the field of menopause. So, many women in the 1970s didn't have access to updated, comprehensive medical information about symptoms, their cause, and how they might be alleviated.

Though your mother may have never discussed menopause with you, that doesn't mean you—and millions of other Baby Boomers—didn't "inherit" certain beliefs about menopause. Your mother's beliefs about menopause and the general attitude of the women in her generation toward this important transition could be transferred to you, whether or not those beliefs were spoken. How your mother handled menopause has likely colored your attitude toward menopause—and will, therefore, help shape your experience.

What Our Mothers Taught Medicine

Since the late 1970s, the medical profession has studied menopausal women more than in any time in history, and what it has learned from those women—a group that includes the mothers of Baby Boomers—has changed the way science and society view menopause. Symptoms such as hot flashes, insomnia, and irritability were viewed as all-in-the-head responses to the panic of aging. Today, many scientists trace these symptoms to specific changes in the body's hormone levels. In the 1980s, most women viewed hormone replacement therapy (HRT) as the only option for relieving menopausal symptoms. Today, HRT is just one treatment choice. The world is a different place for today's menopausal women thanks, in part, to data gathered for and by their mothers' generation.

Today, any woman approaching menopause has a wide variety of health care resources, treatment options, support groups, information sources, and discussion forums to turn to for information, advice, and ideas about having a healthy, satisfying transition to menopause. Menopausal women don't have to "shut up and get through it" or deny that they're experiencing natural emotional and physical reactions to this important passage. Today's fifty-year-olds have one-third of their lives ahead of them. They will live longer than any generation of women that preceded them, and they won't experience this "Third Age" as their mothers experienced it. To live the years ahead productively and happily, women in this group must come face to face with their body, their health, and their attitudes toward making the transition to menopause.

Common Wisdom: What's It Worth?

Do you remember Health Education or Sex Ed classes back in the late 1960s or early 1970s? If so, you undoubtedly recall the plastic model of the female reproductive organs that graced the teacher's desk. At some point in the course, the teacher would send the model around the room, so everyone could get a closer look. The girls would pass the model around, eyeing it casually and handing it to the next student—nothing to see here, folks! The sexual revolution was just unfolding, and young girls were learning to regard their bodies and sexuality in wholly new ways.

In a time of growing sexual freedom, Baby Boomers learned to be cool and nonchalant about sexuality—and they certainly weren't caught up in issues their mothers and grandmothers thought of as "female problems." They laughed at old euphemisms for menstruation, such as "falling off the roof" or "getting the curse." In an age of feminism, these women learned to toss aside the old concepts of feminine weakness and fragility and recognize themselves as strong, capable, freethinking, sexual creatures.

But now, as they approach menopause, many women in this postfeminist age are considering their femaleness from another perspective. At some point, every woman begins to contemplate certain facts about this time of transition, and to acknowledge some of the following basic truths:

- Some physical aspects of the aging process are unique to women;
- The body and mind of a fifty-year-old woman is different from that of a twenty-five-year-old woman;
- Menopause marks a physical change in a woman's body, and every woman's reaction to that physical change will be different.

Beyond these simple, basic truths, however, most of us hold a number of ideas and attitudes toward menopause and aging—some true and some false. So how do you think about menopause? Do you dread it? Are you looking forward to the freedom of moving beyond menstruation and into a life free of the possibility of unwanted pregnancy? Or do you equate fertility with femininity, and worry that menopause will leave you dried up and dreary? Are you hopeful that with the right diet, treatment plan, and nutritional supplements you can get back the body you had at twenty-five? Or at least keep the one you have at forty-five? Do you know the woman you are, and can you accept the woman you are becoming?

Your attitude toward menopause and the aging process will determine the answers to many of these questions. And the first step in understanding how you feel about menopause is to examine the source of those feelings and ideas. The common wisdom of menopause—the information and misinformation that fuels society's beliefs—plays an important role in determining what we believe. We may know that a widely held belief is simply untrue, but it's easier to sort fact from fiction when we take a moment to understand the nugget of truth that may have blossomed into a full-blown myth. So, take a moment to review some of the beliefs that make up the common wisdom of menopause, so you can understand the truths—and untruths—they hold.

Menopausal Women Lose Interest in Sex

The lack-of-libido mythology about women in menopause is part of the common wisdom shared by both men and women—and it's simply not true. Masters and Johnson conducted a study that demonstrated no link between estrogen levels and libido. A number of studies have shown that only a small percentage of postmenopausal women report a lack of interest in sex, and over half of all women studied report no decrease in sexual interest at all after menopause. In fact, the American Association of Retired Persons (AARP) *Modern Maturity* Sexual Survey, conducted in 1999, showed over two-thirds of men and women age forty-five and older say they're satisfied with their sex lives, and many say they enjoy sex "now more than ever."

So where did this myth come from? The truth is that women suffering from severe estrogen depletion can experience some discomfort during sex due to drier, thinner, less flexible vaginal walls and occasional itching and burning near the vaginal opening. A woman experiencing hot flashes, disturbed sleep patterns, headaches, and other occasional symptoms of menopause is unlikely to feel as sexually eager as she would otherwise. However, none of these conditions is permanent or untreatable, and many of them aren't inevitable, either. So, if you believe that menopause equals the end of sex as you know it, you're wrong.

Women in Menopause Gain Weight, Have Hot Flashes, and Lose Control of Their Emotions

Lots of people think that the typical woman in menopause is fat, flushed, and out of control. While hot flashes, weight gain, and mood swings arc all symptoms reported by some women in menopause, they aren't inevitable side effects of the passage. In fact, many women—as many as 10 to 20 percent of women studied—exhibit no symptoms of menopause at all. And while studies show that as many as half of all women in perimenopause experience some weight gain, other women actually lose weight during perimenopause; and many of those who gain weight before menopause lose it afterward. (See Chapters 13 and 14 for information about weight management in menopause.)

Perhaps as many as 85 percent of menopausal women report hot flashes, but most women find them to be intermittent and, on average, they diminish completely within five years after menopause. (See Chapter 16.)

Irritability and depression are also symptoms reported by some—but not all—women during perimenopause, but no one should expect depression to be a long-term, ongoing fact of life during this transition. In fact, depression is reported at much higher rates among women in their twenties and thirties, and some studies have shown that depression actually decreases in postmenopausal women. And even if you do experience mood swings, they don't have to become part of your identity during menopause. (See Chapter 18.)

In short, you may or may not have hot flashes, moodiness, and weight gain during menopause—many women don't. But if you do experience these symptoms they are likely to be temporary and can be treated by a number of therapeutic options.

Hormone Replacement Therapy Is Dangerous

Almost 35 percent of women in menopause use some form of hormone replacement therapy (HRT). It's true that HRT can have dangerous consequences for women with a history of breast cancer, blood clots, endometrial cancer, and certain other family health concerns. No reputable doctor would prescribe HRT for a woman whose health history indicates it may be harmful for her. But most doctors agree that HRT is one of the most effective methods available today for minimizing both the uncomfortable symptoms (such as hot flashes and vaginal dryness) and health-threatening side effects (including elevated cholesterol levels and bone loss) of menopause. Still, many women continue to view HRT as a treatment option pushed by doctors as a means of making money for both the medical profession and the pharmaceutical industry.

Many of the studies that indicated links between estrogen and endometrial cancer were conducted on women who were given estrogen alone, without the balancing hormone progesterone, in the early days of HRT. Today, doctors prescribe both hormones for women who still have a uterus. Women who take both hormones actually have a lower risk of endometrial cancer than women who take no hormones. And other studies show that the benefits of HRT, including reduced heart disease, improved blood cholesterol levels, and lowered incidences of osteoporosis, far outweigh the risks.

ESSENTIALS

Many, many studies on the benefits and potential health implications of HRT are underway, and new reports appear regularly. To keep up with some of the latest news about HRT, you can search under "Menopause" on the National Library of Medicine's Web site at *www.nlm.nih.gov/medlineplus/menopause.html.*

You may or may not be a good candidate for HRT, and you certainly can use other methods for treating symptoms. If you do decide to use HRT, you may take it for only a short period of time. To know and understand your options, read as much as you can on the topic and talk with your doctor and other health care professionals. But keep an open mind, listen to the facts, and learn all you can about HRT. (See Chapter 11 for more information.) Then make your decision based on fact—not fear.

HRT Is the Only Viable Option for Dealing with the Symptoms of Menopause

HRT isn't the only option for treating menopause symptoms or delaying the aging effects of slowing estrogen production. Depending upon the symptoms you experience, simple lifestyle changes may address your most annoying reminders of perimenopause. During your mother's experience with menopause, HRT was just about the only treatment option discussed with women in the transition. So many women in that generation faced an HRT-or-nothing choice. But, the truths of menopause have changed dramatically over the past thirty years.

QUESTIONS?

What exactly are alternative treatments for symptoms of menopause?
Alternative treatments are any treatment other than the traditional treatment of hormone replacement therapy. Alternative treatments include anything from vitamins and herbs, to nutritional supplements of soy and phytoestrogens, to cognitive therapy, acupuncture, and biofeedback.

As women have learned more about the causes and life cycles of certain menopausal symptoms, they feel more comfortable tackling some of them with simple lifestyle changes. You can sleep in a cool bedroom and wear layers of clothing to combat hot flashes, for example. Relaxation therapies can help reduce the occurrence of insomnia, as can changes in eating and drinking habits. If you suffer from anxiety and depression, you might benefit from psychological counseling or biofeedback therapy. A number of herbal remedies, prescription and over-the-counter medications, and dietary supplements are available to help fight off bone loss, high cholesterol, sleeplessness, and other menopause-related health concerns. Women who cannot or prefer not to use estrogen can choose from a number of sound, viable non-HRT treatment options for combating the symptoms of menopause.

Menopausal Women Are Angry, Bitter, and Old

You need only to look around you to see through this lie. First, the average age of menopause in the United States is fifty-one—hardly an age that anyone in today's society (anyone over the age of twenty) would view as being old. And some women go through menopause—even natural menopause—in their forties. There's a big difference between growing older and being "old." And who has time to be hung up on chronology, anyway? It's how old you *feel* that counts.

Beyond that, few women in this society have lives that grind to a halt when their reproductive system slows down. Women's lives aren't defined by the number of children sitting around their supper table each evening, and the empty nest more often than not evolves into a house full of other interests and opportunities. Many women are just entering the most productive and lucrative stages of their careers during and after menopause, and find that their career satisfaction actually increases at this time. Menopause can be a time of unprecedented self-confidence, freedom, and financial liberation for women. Anger and bitterness aren't a natural and inevitable side effect of the transition.

Menopause is a time of reflection, though. For many women, menopause is a time of introspection and personal assessment. Some women have spent the majority of their lives preceding menopause caring for other people and interests—children, spouses or partners, parents, and careers. If these women turn more attention inward, their behavior might on the surface make them appear to be withdrawn or even angry. Menopause is a time of change, and for many women that change extends deeper than the rhythm of their ovarian cycles. Blanket assumptions about the feelings and attitudes of menopausal women—or women of any age, for that matter—are never accurate.

Constructing Your Own Common Wisdom

The previous sections discuss only a few of the commonly held misconceptions about the experience of perimenopause and menopause. While these examples help illustrate how wrong these generalities can be, many other inaccuracies dominate the popular culture about menopause and what it means to go through it. Common wisdom exists because it's easier to accept a set of broad generalizations than it is to dig out the facts of any issue or idea. But when it comes to the subject of menopause, generalities that apply in the majority of cases simply don't exist. Every woman's experience in menopause will differ. And yours is really the only experience that matters to you. If you keep an open mind and pay attention to your own body and the facts about menopause it teaches you, you'll find your own set of common wisdom truths about this transition and what it means for you. If you monitor and respond to your own body's reactions, and discuss your concerns openly and thoroughly with your health care provider, you'll be better able to make the best lifestyle and health care decisions for you during your passage through menopause.

Your Chances for a Brand New Start

If women in the past thought of menopause as the beginning of the end, more and more women today are seizing upon this time of transition as an opportunity to make important changes in their lifestyles and behavior. As mentioned earlier, many women devote their premenopausal adult years to focusing outward, on the demands of family, finances, and careers. As a woman approaches menopause, however, her life may offer her many new opportunities for personal freedom and growth. Many postmenopausal women find that their families and home life actually improves at this time and that they have a greater sense of personal fulfillment.

With less time spent caring for young children, or developing first-time relationships with husbands or partners, or gaining a foothold in the workplace, postmenopausal women can devote more time to their personal interests. Women find new energy and interest in returning to pursuits they abandoned in their twenties and thirties, including creative outlets such as painting, writing, and photography. Many women at the age of menopause find themselves able to devote time and energy to travel, finishing an abandoned academic degree, or starting a new business.

Menopause is a time when many women make important lifestyle changes. During most of your life, you may not have worried much about issues such as nutrition and exercise or the health-threatening impact of smoking, living with stress, or inadequate sleep. But as you approach the age of menopause, you may find that you're ready to make changes in your habits now, in order to ensure a happier, healthy future. In fact, though the stereotype of age may be that it's a time of reminiscence and living in the past, many women find themselves contemplating the future more than ever as they approach menopause. Though you may be nearing the end of your reproductive years, your productivity may achieve levels you've never known.

Part of the freedom of menopause is that it gives women an opportunity to define themselves in terms of who they are, rather than how well they fit the stereotype of what women can be. Many women spend their youth attempting to fulfill the popular culture's ideal of what a woman should be: thin, beautiful, neat, industrious, helpful, tireless, and supportive of family, friends, supervisor, parents, and anyone else that she encounters in her day. In other words, she's a mother, a wife, and a helper. Women in menopause have an opportunity to throw down that identity and discover what they want, what they enjoy, and how they can best fulfill their needs.

In her book *The Wisdom of Menopause*, Dr. Christiane Northrup stresses that most menopausal women do grieve past losses. When you're no longer a young mother, a young wife, or a "fresh, young face" at the office, you realize that one identity is passing, even as another begins. But Dr. Northrup contends that the biggest message menopause brings women is not one of loss; rather, menopause is a wake-up call, "as each woman struggles to make a new life, one that can accommodate her emerging self."

Since you were born, you have been in a constant state of growth and change. Through the years, your attitudes and beliefs have helped determine how well you fared in each stage of your life. Your ability to adapt to change, to take advantage of opportunities that came your way, and to capitalize on the realities of your situation have determined the successes or failures you've enjoyed—in both your personal and professional lives. That's why your attitudes and beliefs about menopause matter. As part of the largest generation of postfifty-year-old women in our nation's history, you have the opportunity to help shape the common wisdom about what postmenopausal women are all about. Deciding to be well-informed and active in the maintenance of your future health and happiness is the surest way toward a good experience with menopause and a healthy, fulfilling postmenopausal life.

Don't imagine that healthy introspection has to lead to an it's-all-about-me attitude. There's a big difference between self-evaluation and self-absorption. Instead, think of your Third Age as an opportunity to become reacquainted with yourself—who you are and what your dreams are, now. This time of self-realization and discovery can benefit both you and your relationships with others.

CHAPTER 5

Working with Your Doctor

In an age of HMOs, PPOs, and a never-ending list of traditional and alternative health care provider options, few women go through their adult lives with a single practitioner. The increased mobility of modern life has served to do away with the lifetime family doctor, too. That's why it's important for every woman to become an active member of her health care "plan" by working closely with her primary care provider.

Do You Have the Doctor You Need Now?

The chance that you'll see the same health care professional at age fifty that you saw at age twenty grows slimmer with each passing day. With the ever-changing parade of health care workers we see over the course of our lives, it becomes easy to think of them as interchangeable cogs in the vast machine of our professional health care maintenance. But that's a dangerous attitude to have toward the individuals responsible for helping you live a long, healthy life.

Your choice of a health care professional must always meet certain qualifications in training and ability—you should never accept second-rate health care, no matter how simple your health care needs may be. But when you're approaching menopause, you require some special qualities in a health care provider. You need to be an active partner in your health maintenance throughout your life; if you have been a passive patient up to this point, now's the time to get serious and get involved in ensuring your good health throughout menopause—and beyond.

QUESTIONS?

Can't my primary care physician handle my health care during menopause?
If both you and your primary care physician (PCP) are comfortable with that arrangement, there's no reason for you to see a specialist during menopause. If you have severe or unusual symptoms, however, your PCP is likely to refer you to a specialist for diagnosis and treatment. Talk to your PCP about his or her recommendations for your health care during menopause.

During perimenopause and menopause, your health care needs differ from those when you were younger. You may begin experiencing abnormalities in your menstrual cycle, such as irregular or heavy bleeding. Your symptoms could be caused by hormonal fluctuations of approaching menopause—or by serious diseases, such as precancerous changes in the lining of the uterus or even endometrial cancer. You may need diagnosis and treatment of emotional as well as physical symptoms. And you most certainly will need the medical advice of someone who is up-to-date on medical advancements in menopause symptoms and treatment, knowledgeable about a range of treatment options, and willing and able to discuss those options with you. Even if you've been pretty casual about health care during your twenties, thirties, and early forties, the approach of menopause signals an end to ho-hum health care. Your health care actions and choices now can determine the quality of the rest of your life.

You may have a great health care provider right now, or you may need to begin your search for the doctor that's right for you. In either case, now is the time to evaluate what you want and need in a health care provider, and to make sure that you have the man or woman that fulfills that role.

Personal Qualities of Your Health Care Provider

When you're choosing a health care provider to give you the medical oversight and guidance you need during menopause, you need to consider a number of qualities. Medical or professional licensing and board certification are a must, of course, but beyond that threshold, what qualities matter most to you in a health care professional? Maybe up to this point, you've been very comfortable with the gruff, no-nonsense doctor who tells you, "This is what you need to do, now go do it," and moves on. Now, however, you may need a doctor who's willing to listen to your fears, questions, and concerns, and who will encourage you to take an active role in managing your health care options. Or maybe you've been perfectly content with the catch-as-catch-can variability of health care service provided by a large local clinic or service, but now you want to establish a real relationship with a doctor and start getting more personalized, in-depth health care testing and treatment. How do you go about deciding what you need your doctor to do—or be?

The first step in choosing the right health care provider for your menopause journey is to determine what kind of person you want to work with.

Ask yourself these questions:

- Do you prefer to see a male or a female health care professional? You're going to need to be comfortable with this person, so you need to decide if gender plays a role in your willingness to discuss symptoms, lifestyle factors, and treatment alternatives. If you'll feel reluctant to be totally open and honest with a health care provider because of his or her gender, this may not be the time to try to break down those barriers.

- Do you feel comfortable with a medical "boss" who will dispense advice and guidance without requesting your input regarding treatment options? Or would you prefer someone who is open to the patient-as-partner approach to health care? There's nothing wrong with expecting your health care provider to suggest specific treatment options—as long as that person is fully trained and has a complete understanding of your medical background and family history. If, on the other hand, you want to discuss and choose from a range of options, you need to be certain that your health care provider is willing to discuss those options with you, and support your decision with good follow-through treatment.

- Do you care about the age of your health care worker? Again, it's important that you feel comfortable with your health care provider, you're willing to openly discuss your health and lifestyle issues, and you're confident in the decisions and recommendations that you're offered.

ESSENTIALS

While personal qualities don't determine a health care professional's skill or training, they may influence the way you work with the person you choose. In the end, you might choose someone who doesn't fit your optimum personality profile, but acknowledging your preferences can help you form a strong working relationship with any health care professional.

Professional Qualifications

Personal qualities aside, the most important factor in your choice of a health care provider should be professional training. When you're choosing medical care specifically for your treatment during menopause, you need first to decide what kind of special training you want your caregiver to have. If you want someone with specialization beyond that of a general practitioner (GP), you can choose from among a number of types of traditional and nontraditional health care providers. Within the realm of traditional medicine, here are some of your choices:

- An obstetrician/gynecologist (ob/gyn) is specially trained in prenatal care for expectant mothers and the delivery of babies (the obstetrician part) and care of women's reproductive health from menarche to menopause and beyond (the gynecologist services). These physicians can provide long-term treatment for women at any development stage or age. You can also choose an ob/gyn with a specialization in menopause. With the menopausal population booming, more ob/gyns are specializing in menopause. These specialists remain up-to-date on menopause symptoms, testing, and treatment methods, and new developments in the use of HRT.
- A reproductive endocrinologist is a doctor who specializes in hormone imbalances and infertility. Since these physicians focus on reproductive hormones, they are likely to remain current on HRT and other treatments and issues that impact menopausal women. Some of these physicians deal strictly with infertility issues, so check before you make the appointment.
- A nurse practitioner is a Registered Nurse (RN) who can perform physical examinations, diagnose and treat illnesses and injuries, prescribe medication, and provide other health care functions. A women's health nurse practitioner (WHNP) has special training in the area of women's health. Recent studies have shown that many people of both sexes are choosing nurse practitioners as primary health care providers, citing satisfaction with such factors as the amount of time spent in discussing health issues and accessibility to patients.

Alternative health care is big business in the United States. A 1997 survey reported in the *Journal of the American Medical Association* (JAMA) revealed that 40 percent of residents of the United States used alternative medicine in 1997 and made over 629 million visits to alternative health care providers that year (as opposed to 386 million visits to primary care physicians). Many women turn to alternative health care techniques during menopause; here are some of the types of health care providers they choose:

"Natural" doesn't mean "safe." Though you can purchase many over-the-counter herbal supplements for relief of menopausal symptoms, you need to be very careful in their use. Many plants and herbs deliver significant doses of estrogen or interact with other supplements and prescription drugs. Check with your doctor or health care provider before embarking on any type of treatment.

- Herbalists prescribe herbal supplements and treatments to combat symptoms of menopause. Herbal remedies are growing in popularity in Western cultures, and many women today turn to herbs such as black cohosh, evening primrose, and gingko biloba to offset symptoms such as hot flashes, insomnia, and memory loss. Herbal substances are not benign treatment alternatives, however, and herbalists are trained to help determine the best types, amounts, and delivery mechanisms for herbal treatment of menopause symptoms.
- Homeopaths offer a type of medical treatment that operates on the principle that like cures like. Homeopaths prescribe small doses of substances that, if not diluted, would actually make symptoms worse; homeopathic prescription amounts are based on the severity of symptoms, rather than the age and weight of the patient.
- Acupuncturists use a 2,000-year-old treatment technique that involves rotating fine, sterilized needles into the patient's skin to bring about a therapeutic response. Many women in menopause turn to acupuncture for relief of such symptoms as headache, anxiety, insomnia, and fatigue.

Mentioned here are just a few types of nontraditional health care providers you might consult during menopause. For a more complete discussion of alternative treatments for symptoms of menopause, see Chapter 12. Many women use alternative medicine techniques to combat symptoms of menopause in conjunction with traditional medical health care. If you're interested in exploring both traditional and alternative medical approaches to treating your menopause symptoms, make sure any health care provider you choose is open to helping you as you pursue this approach.

Finding the Right Fit

When you determine what kind of health care professional you want, you have a number of options for finding someone in your area whose qualifications match your needs. Here are just a few ways you can locate a health care provider:

- Ask your GP or family physician. He or she may know who of the qualified individuals in your area have approaches and skills suitable for the type of health care assistance you're looking for. Since this person knows your style and personality, he or she may be able to match you with someone that's right for you.
- Ask your family and friends. Though the practitioner that's best for them may not be the one for you, the women you know can give you an inside perspective on their health care providers. Coworkers may also be able to suggest a physician that is convenient, in terms of proximity to your workplace or association with a nearby hospital. And since your coworkers may be on the same insurance plan that you have, they might be able to help you anticipate—or even avoid—problems with insurance filing.
- Visit the NAMS (North American Menopause Society) Web site at *www.menopause.org* to download a list of health care providers registered with the Society as menopause specialists. The listing indicates licensing and location to help you narrow your search in these key areas.

- Call reputable medical clinics in your area to find out if their services include a menopause clinic or specialists.
- Check with your insurance provider to see if it offers a list of doctors and therapists with menopause specialties. Most health insurance companies have Web sites listing physicians in your area or affiliated with major hospitals.
- Go online. You can search for menopause specialists in your area using any of the major search engines such as Google, Northern Light, or Excite.

When you've narrowed the list of potential health care providers, your search has just begun. Now, you need to dig into each health care provider's operation to find out how well it meshes with your needs and preferences. Follow a few practical guidelines for screening health care provider candidates:

- Call the office, and pay attention to the details of your experience. Is the office big and busy or small and personal? Are you immediately put on hold, and if so, how long do you wait? Can the receptionist answer your questions or put you in contact with someone who can? What are the office hours? How does the doctor or practitioner handle emergency calls? How long will it take for you to get an appointment? What's the length of an average office visit—you want to make sure you have adequate time with the doctor or practitioner during your visit. Can patients get responses to questions over the telephone or through e-mail? If so, who returns those calls or e-mails?
- Make sure you find out what kinds of insurance the office accepts, and how insurance billing is handled. You'll also want to check with your insurance provider to be certain that any alternative or specialty treatment you receive is covered before you embark on any potentially expensive testing or treatment plan.
- Try to schedule an information visit with the doctor or practitioner, then use that visit to assess the condition of the office, the helpfulness of the staff, and your impression of the health care provider. If the doctor or practitioner doesn't limit his or her practice

to menopause (and most don't), find out approximately what percentage of the patient load involves menopause treatment.

- Find out if the practice has a person—such as an office manager or assistant to the primary health care provider—who can answer your questions and help you get the service you need when the doctor or practitioner is busy or away from the office. Some offices have a registered nurse who performs this function, while others use a medical assistant or even a layperson with extensive medical knowledge and training. The title isn't as important as this individual's willingness and ability to help you resolve issues satisfactorily.

FACTS

Your health care provider will have a big impact on the decisions you make about therapies and treatment. In one study by a medical researcher from the Harvard Medical School, 96 percent of women in an HMO who had received an initial prescription for HRT cited their doctor's opinion as critical to their decision to pursue that treatment option.

Your prescreening efforts are well worth the time and effort you invest in them. The health care provider you choose will be an important part of your life for several years to come. Choosing the provider who works best for you can make all of your health care decisions easier and help ensure that you get the best available care, advice, and guidance.

Talk with Your Doctor

Finding a great doctor or other health care provider is only half of the sound menopause management equation. In order to make the best decisions and follow the best lifestyle decisions and treatment approaches, you need to be an active, informed, involved partner in your health care program. You're reading this book, which indicates that you understand the importance of becoming well informed about menopause issues, symptoms, and treatment options. Use the information you read here (and in the recommended resources listed in Appendix B) to decide what kinds of questions and options you want to explore with your health care provider. The following sections discuss some simple ways you can prepare to be a good patient who brings out the best in her good doctor.

If you're seeing a doctor or practitioner about issues related to menopause, you aren't a kid anymore. As obvious as that seems, it's important that you drop a lot of the passive techniques you may have developed when dealing with doctors (and other authority figures) in your youth. If you've followed the advice given up to this point in the chapter, you've spent a lot of time and energy tracking down the right doctor or practitioner to help you deal most effectively with the symptoms and biological and physiological effects of menopause. So do your health care provider a favor, and approach your consultation as an exchange of information—not a tell-me-what-to-do-and-I'll-leave event.

During your initial office visit, the doctor or practitioner will ask you a number of questions regarding your individual and family health histories. As a rule, you'll need to report on any personal and family history of blood clots, heart disease, breast cancer, and osteoporosis, among other conditions. Your doctor or practitioner will also ask you about your current medications—both over-the-counter and prescription drugs—as well as your use of alcohol, recreational drugs, and tobacco. You're not running for class president here, so don't attempt to whitewash the facts by presenting yourself as you think you should be. If you drink or smoke, say so. And don't forget that over-the-counter medications such as pain relievers, vitamins, minerals, and nutritional supplements count; report any substances you regularly consume, so your doctor or practitioner can be aware of them when he or she prescribes treatment.

ESSENTIALS

When you're visiting your menopause specialist, tell it like it is—don't exaggerate or downplay the symptoms you've experienced. Your caregiver needs to understand the full range and severity of your symptoms. You can't get the best health care treatment if you aren't completely honest when describing your condition.

During your first visit, remember to mention all symptoms you've been experiencing—both emotional and physical. If your periods have become irregular in any way, report the irregularities. (Take your menstrual calendar to the visit.) Mood swings and depression are important indicators of your current health, as is any change in your interest in sex. If you're suffering from periodic involuntary urine release, report that and explain the conditions. Take a written list of symptoms, questions, and concerns with you to your visit, and write down the answers you receive.

ESSENTIALS

If you've been keeping a menstruation journal or menstrual calendar (see Chapter 3), take it to your initial visit with your menopause specialist. Your doctor or practitioner can gain valuable information about your current condition by reviewing even a two- or three-month history of your symptoms. Add to your calendar any symptoms that seem to run in cycles, such as headaches, water retention, or unusual pelvic pain.

Before you leave the office, make sure you understand all of the information you've received during your visit. If you need further explanation, ask for it. You won't get points for pretending to understand information that confuses you. If your doctor or practitioner is using terminology you don't understand, ask for a translation. Asking for clarification immediately is preferable to calling the office after you've returned home to report that you didn't understand something you were told during your visit. Many doctors' offices also have preprinted brochures regarding various aspects of menopause, so feel free to ask.

Finally, discuss all treatment options that interest you, regardless of the medical specialization of the health care provider you've chosen. If you're interested in pursuing a combination approach to managing symptoms of menopause, you want to be certain that this doctor or practitioner is open to that approach. If you are looking for relief from specific symptoms, such as incontinence or insomnia, say so, and ask if any recommended treatment options specifically address those symptoms. If you think you may want certain tests that the doctor hasn't actually offered, speak up. If you have insurance coverage issues, bring this up as well. The more you understand about the specific functions and goals of treatment programs, the better able you'll be to decide which plan is right for you (and the more likely you'll be to follow the plan as recommended).

Take an Active Role

In order for any therapy to be effective, you must be committed to following it—as directed—for as long as is necessary to gauge its results and effectiveness. Remember, you aren't a passive observer in your journey through menopause. Being an active partner in your treatment plan involves carefully monitoring your response to therapeutic drugs and treatments, and keeping your health care provider(s) informed of your progress. If you have a negative reaction to drugs or other treatment options, speak up. You could be experiencing normal adjustment reactions or you could be embarking on a plan that simply doesn't match your body chemistry, lifestyle, or biological and physiological makeup. You won't know what's wrong unless you report the reaction to your doctor or practitioner.

If you are using a combination of treatment options, make sure that you coordinate all of them with your primary caregiver. Maybe you've heard about the benefits of using biofeedback-assisted behavioral training to control urine discharge, and you'd like to explore that option. Before you contact a psychologist, physical therapist, or clinician to schedule a biofeedback session, talk to your menopause specialist about the process, to make sure biofeedback won't conflict with other treatment plans you're pursuing. Seeking a second opinion is fine, and often is a good idea; but remember to reflect on all the options you have been offered, and consult the specialist you feel most comfortable with about combining therapies.

Finally, don't remain passively disappointed with your treatment. If you feel unhappy with the health care you're receiving, just say so. Your doctor, practitioner, or therapist can't correct a problem that he or she doesn't know about. If you're unhappy with the progress of your symptom-relief treatment, discuss your concerns with your menopause specialist. If you feel that your doctor or practitioner is unresponsive to your questions and concerns, give him or her an opportunity to discuss your feelings. Although you want to build and maintain a respectful relationship with your caregiver, choose honesty over diplomacy in this discussion. Be very specific and open as you state your concerns, and listen carefully to your caregiver's response. If you can't resolve your differences, it's time to start looking for another health care partner.

Don't judge the quality of your menopause specialist by how often that person agrees with you. You want a health care provider who'll help you pursue a treatment path that's effective and safe. Find someone you can trust, then discuss your concerns and ideas with an open mind, and—if necessary—seek a second or third opinion.

Instructions for putting together your postforty health management plan appear in the following chapter. But for now, it's important to remember that active, involved follow-through is a critical component of any treatment and lifestyle plan you adopt.

Listen Up, Speak Up, Be Honest

Throughout this chapter, you're reminded that you carry a big part of the responsibility for making sure that you get the best possible health care. When you've chosen a health care provider that meets your needs and fits your own list of qualifications, you can't simply sit back and enjoy the ride. To make sure that you help your health care provider continue to give you the best advice and treatment options during your transition through perimenopause, remember the following important guidelines:

- Listen to the information your health care provider gives you. When you ask a question, take notes of the response if necessary; don't assume that you already know what your caregiver is going to say. Just listen carefully, and ask further questions, if necessary.

- Ask questions, voice concerns, report problems, and discuss options; your caregiver depends upon your active involvement in your health care plan.

- Be honest. You must be honest in your communications with your health care provider. Many people think that they'll annoy their doctor or health care provider by asking too many questions or by discussing issues that they don't fully understand or agree with. Most doctors and other health care providers find it much more challenging to deal with patients who act as though they're okay with a plan or fully understand a treatment option, when that isn't really the case. You can't have a good health care experience if you don't communicate honestly with your health care provider.

CHAPTER 6

General Health Risks and Management after Age Forty

If the first forty years of your life were spent in blissful ignorance of the toll that each passing year might take on your physical health, now is the time to get serious about your personal maintenance plan. If you are aware of the common health risks women face after forty, you will know what changes you need to make in your diet and lifestyle.

The Health Risks We Face after Forty

First, let's all agree that age isn't a number, and turning forty doesn't signal an onslaught of health-riddling diseases and disabilities. Many women are healthier than they've ever been as they approach midlife. But a well-thought-out approach to health management and maintenance is smart at any age, and it becomes more important as each year passes. Don't think of your health care efforts as part of entering old age; think of them as a simple, basic plan to preserve and extend your youth.

Everyone—man and woman—has to invest a bit more time and attention in his or her "machine" as it ages. Our bodies work hard, and after years of service, even routine maintenance becomes more demanding—and essential. If we reach a stage where our jobs and personal lives have become less physically demanding but, perhaps, more mentally draining, it's easy to overlook the shifting load our bodies must bear. We lose track of the tradeoffs we've made in how we spend our time and mental energy with less time spent outdoors and in fewer physical activities, and more time spent sitting behind desks or in the car, struggling to meet deadlines, resolving problems, or sorting out schedules. Many people enter their forties sandwiched between caring for their children and parents at the same time. Add to that the accumulation of many years of not-so-healthy habits—basing our nutrition pyramid on sugar, fat, and deep-fried anything; smoking; yo-yo-ing from one weight-loss plan to the next; skimping on sleep, then counting on caffeine to power us through the day—and it's easy to see why our bodies might need a little TLC as they hit midlife.

For women, though, the physical effects of an aging reproductive system can present some special health risks. Estrogen provides women with a natural protection against certain diseases, such as osteoporosis, heart disease, and vaginal atrophy. In perimenopause, because a woman's body produces less estrogen, she becomes more vulnerable to these and other health risks. Many physical symptoms that might be attributed to the first pangs of aging might actually be the first warning signals of serious health problems in the making. So a good health care regimen at age forty can lay the groundwork for a healthy passage through ages fifty, sixty, seventy, eighty, and beyond.

The following sections of this chapter look at some of the most common age-related health factors that deserve your attention as you approach menopause. When you understand the types of health risks and issues you may face, you can begin sketching the outline of your own midlife health management strategy. The "Your After-Forty Health Maintenance Plan" section of this chapter offers you smart detection and prevention methods that can help you manage these risks as you move toward and through menopause.

FACTS

Many women view breast cancer as their greatest health threat, but heart disease is a much greater risk for women. According to the American Heart Association, nearly twice as many women in the United States die of heart disease and stroke than from all forms of cancer combined—and that includes breast cancer.

Heart Disease and Menopause

Heart disease is a term we've all heard, but may not fully understand. The umbrella term covers a wide range of diseases, illnesses, and events that impact the heart and circulatory system—known as cardiovascular diseases. High blood pressure and coronary artery disease that can lead to stroke, heart attacks, and early death are some of the most common forms of heart disease for both men and women.

We've all grown accustomed to thinking of the typical victim of heart disease as a middle-aged, overweight, out-of-shape man, but that's yet another stereotype that just doesn't reflect the real picture. Heart disease is the number one killer of women over fifty in America today—or, putting it another way, one out of two women will die of cardiovascular disease. According to the Women's Health Network, over 500,000 women may die of heart disease in this country in 2002. It's true that prior to menopause women suffer fewer effects of heart disease and stroke than men. But as women age, their risk of heart disease increases dramatically. More than half of all stroke deaths occur in women.

Some studies indicate that a woman's natural estrogen loss due to aging may contribute to heart disease. Estrogen can help control the body's blood cholesterol levels, and it keeps a woman's total cholesterol low before menopause, with low levels of LDL (low-density lipoproteins or "bad" cholesterol) and high levels of the "good" cholesterol, HDL (high-density lipoproteins). These fractions are reversed after menopause, and are thought to be serious contributors to one's risk of a heart attack. Women over age fifty-five have higher blood cholesterol levels than men, and women are particularly vulnerable to low levels of HDL.

FACTS

If you're courting obesity and high cholesterol, you're speeding up the effects of age on your heart's health. According to the American Heart Association's 2001 Heart and Stroke Statistical Update, nearly 34 percent of the average diet in the United States is made up of fat and over half of all Americans have high blood total cholesterol levels (over 200 mg/dl).

Estrogen loss isn't the only contributing factor to heart disease and stroke for women as they move through perimenopause, however. If as you approach menopause you begin putting on weight, particularly around your abdomen (starting to look like an "apple" instead of a "pear"), you could be significantly increasing your risk of heart disease. Other midlife diseases, such as diabetes and high blood pressure, are heavily linked to the onset of heart disease in midlife, as well.

Too often, heart attacks are misdiagnosed in women with the symptoms attributed to heartburn, indigestion, or gallbladder disease. As women move toward menopause, their risk factors for heart disease increase dramatically, and so their vigilance and heart-healthy habits have to increase to offset the risk. Although family health history plays a role in your own likelihood of developing heart disease, you have many options for combating this deadly enemy, including diet, exercise, lifestyle changes, cholesterol-controlling medications, HRT, and more.

Cancer Risks

Though heart disease is a more common disease among American women, cancer is one of the most feared. Cancer is the second leading cause of death in the United States; nearly four of every ten Americans will have some kind of cancer at some point during their lives, and nearly 80 percent of those diagnosed with cancer are age fifty-five or older. One-third of all women in the United States will develop cancer during their lifetimes, so as you approach menopause, it's important that you understand which cancers have age-related risk factors for women.

Cancer isn't one disease. Actually cancer is a family of diseases, all of which occur when cell growth goes out of control in some part of the body. Cancer has been widely studied, but its causes are complex and still not fully understood. Contributing factors include environmental pollutants, heredity, occupation, nutrition, and lifestyle. At times, there is no medical explanation for why a certain type of cancer develops in a previously healthy person. Different cancers produce very different illnesses, each with its own symptoms, causes, and risk factors. The following sections discuss some of the most common cancers women face as they move into middle age. The object of this information isn't to alarm you or to convince you that you're doomed to suffer from this disease. But knowledge is power; this brief overview gives you a heads up to the risks your health management plan should monitor.

#1 Cancer Threat for Women: Lung Cancer

Lung cancer is the leading cause of cancer death for women in the United States, and tobacco smoke is the leading cause of lung cancer. The American Lung Association reports that nearly 68,000 women died in the United States from lung cancer in 2000, as opposed to 41,000 who died from breast cancer. Though neither menopause nor age is a contributing factor in this disease, most women are diagnosed with lung cancer at age fifty—right around the time they hit menopause, and often after thirty-five or more years of tobacco smoke exposure. Women are twice as likely as men to contract cancer from tobacco smoke, including secondhand smoke—the vast majority of nonsmokers who contract lung cancer are women.

ESSENTIALS

Since 1950, lung cancer deaths in women in the United States have increased by a startling 600 percent. Every woman smoker knows she should quit, but many fear weight gain, anxiety, and unquenchable cravings during withdrawal. Don't be afraid; you have more options for quitting now than ever before, including patches, gum, medications, and hypnosis. Do whatever it takes to quit now.

If you're approaching menopause, the time is right for you to quit smoking—now. You're approaching a new phase of your life, so why not start it smoke-free? Smoking increases your chances of contracting cervical cancer, emphysema, and other life-threatening chronic lung conditions. Any illness you contract will be complicated by the effects of smoking. Smoking is a sure way to derail an active, healthy passage into middle life.

Don't think for a minute that it's too late to matter; quitting smoking can give you health benefits right away. According to the American Cancer Society (ACS), within twenty minutes after you quit, your body starts regenerating and your blood pressure begins to return to normal. Within eight hours, the carbon monoxide level in your blood drops to normal. Twenty-four hours after you quit, your chance of heart attack begins to decrease. One to nine months later, you should lose that smoker's cough and the sinus congestion, fatigue, and shortness of breath smokers suffer. Within ten years of quitting, you will have cut your risk of lung-cancer death in half; after fifteen years, your chance of contracting coronary heart disease is the same as that of a nonsmoker.

A L E R T

Don't go it alone! You may double your chances of success if you use nicotine replacement, join a stop-smoking class, use a self-help book, or try some other means of smoking cessation support. Visit the American Cancer Society's Web site at *www.cancer.org*, or call them at 1-800-ACS-2345 for help with your efforts.

#2 Cancer Threat for Women: Breast Cancer

Breast cancer is the second most common form of cancer contracted by women today, and advancing age appears to be a major risk factor in its development. Nearly 80 percent of all breast cancers are found in women over fifty, and the incidence of diagnosis and fatality both seem to rise with age. The American Cancer Society (ACS) reports that 163 per 100,000 women in the United States in their forties are diagnosed with breast cancer each year, and twenty-nine die of it; 374 per 100,000 women in their sixties will be diagnosed, and ninety of those will die from the disease. Age isn't the sole risk factor; heredity, lifestyle, family health history, and personal health history, including early menstruation (before age twelve) and late menopause (after fifty-five), all can have an impact on your likelihood of developing breast cancer.

If your mother, sister, or daughter has had breast cancer, your risks of contracting it go up two to three times (depending on how many of these first degree relatives are involved). And, if you've had breast cancer before, you have a higher risk of developing it again. If you've never had a child, or had your first child after age thirty, your risk goes up as well. But what about risk factors that you can change? The American Cancer Society lists the following risk factors for breast cancer that are specifically linked to lifestyle choices:

Hormone replacement therapy (HRT): Most large studies and most world experts agree that long-term use of estrogen after menopause does not increase your risk of breast cancer. However, according to the ACS, a very few studies suggest that long-term use (ten or more years) of HRT may result in a slight increase in the risk of breast cancer. These conflicting studies have not gone unnoticed, and the connection between breast cancer and HRT is still the subject of ongoing research. Some medical professionals suspect that women who take estrogen are more likely to do self-breast exams, see their physicians regularly, and have mammograms. These women are more likely to have their cancers diagnosed at a very early stage, usually before they can even be palpated by the physician or on a self-breast exam, so these tiny cancers can be cured with conservative surgery such as lumpectomy. These women also live longer than their counterparts who take no hormones, presumably due to their regular medical checkups and the protective effect of estrogen on the heart.

Alcohol: Women who have one alcoholic drink a day have a slightly increased risk of contracting breast cancer; two to five drinks daily can up your risk to one and one-half times that of nondrinkers.

Diet: The connection between obesity and breast cancer risk is still being studied, but research indicates that after menopause, your risk of contracting breast cancer is greater if you are overweight. How much of this risk is linked to your body fat versus specific dietary fat content is still under debate. Another issue may be that more breast tissue (obese women tend to have bigger breasts) makes it harder to find an early, small cancerous lump, both on exam and on mammogram.

Exercise: Although research has begun only recently, early findings reported by the ACS seem to indicate that even moderate physical activity can lower breast cancer risk. And maintaining good overall physical condition certainly improves your chances of having fewer complications related to medical and surgical treatment for any disease—including breast cancer.

Survival rates for breast cancer are highest when the cancer is detected early. The five-year survival rate (your chance of being alive five years after the diagnosis of cancer is made) is 96 percent for women whose cancer is caught at an early stage. Early detection helps keep the surgery or other treatment that follows diagnosis as noninvasive and conservative as is possible. Techniques for incorporating breast cancer detection into your general health maintenance plan appear later in this chapter.

Endometrial and Ovarian Cancers

In the United States, cancer of the endometrium—the lining of the uterus—is the most common cancer of the female reproductive organs. The ACS expected that over 36,000 new cases of endometrial cancer would be diagnosed in the United States during 2001; this cancer has a five-year survival rate of about 84 percent.

Your risk of developing endometrial cancer increases as you age. The average age of diagnosis for this cancer is sixty, and 95 percent of all endometrial cancer occurs in women age forty or older.

FACTS

Endometrial cancer is usually preceded by a precancerous condition called endometrial hyperplasia, which is easily diagnosed with a test—endometrial biopsy—that your physician can perform in the office. This test takes about one minute, requires no anesthesia or sedation, and produces very reliable results.

A number of risk factors can contribute to the development of endometrial cancer:

Total number of years of menstruation: Your body's total lifetime exposure to estrogen, without the balancing hormone progesterone, can have an impact on your likelihood of developing endometrial cancer. If you began having periods at a young age (such as before the age of twelve or eleven), continued having periods past age fifty, and have had few or no children (which gives your body a break from the constant estrogen production), your ovaries have been producing estrogen for a greater number of years than the average woman. The more estrogen (and less progesterone) your body has experienced over the years, the higher your risk of developing endometrial cancer.

Obesity: Depending upon how obese you are, your excess body fat can increase your chances of developing endometrial cancer two to five times. Body fat can convert other hormones into estrogen, and having excess body fat contributes to a woman's estrogen levels—and risks of developing this cancer. Diets high in animal fats also may contribute to this risk factor, as can diabetes—a disease common among obese women. Women who are overweight are also more likely to have abnormal menstrual periods, because their ovaries fail to ovulate—thus not producing enough progesterone, in relation to their estrogen. (See "The Phases of Menstruation" in Chapter 3.)

Estrogen replacement therapy (ERT): ERT—hormone therapy that doesn't include progesterone—can increase a woman's chance of developing endometrial cancer. Though doctors used to prescribe ERT for relief from hot flashes, osteoporosis, and heart disease, today doctors almost exclusively combine estrogen with progesterone in HRT, which eliminates the increased risk of endometrial cancer. Of course, if you have had a hysterectomy, you do not need a prescription for progesterone added to your estrogen, since your risk of endometrial cancer is zero.

If you have had breast or ovarian cancer, you may have an increased risk for developing endometrial cancer. Some of the same risk factors contribute to all of these forms of cancer, so with the diagnosis of one, your physician will also monitor you closely for these other cancer types.

If endometrial cancer is diagnosed early, it has an excellent survival rate. Precancerous changes, such as endometrial hyperplasia, often become known through unusual spotting, bleeding, or discharge. Often, these symptoms are apparent for years before actual cancer develops. Sometimes women have had irregular periods for their entire lives, and forget to report this to their health care practitioner. Besides, when you're entering menopause, irregular bleeding, spotting, and discharges aren't supposed to be unusual occurrences at all, so how do you know when to worry that your irregularity is signaling endometrial cancer?

Unfortunately, Pap smears—which are great at detecting cervical cancer—don't reveal endometrial cancer. And many women assume that a normal Pap smear is an assurance of perfect gynecologic health. The best way to stay on top of this and other risks is to provide your health caregiver with a complete family and personal health history, so he or she can best monitor your health. Unless you're at high risk for developing this disease, your doctor won't run yearly detection tests.

However, if you suffer from unusual bleeding that lasts more than two weeks, consult your doctor right away—no matter what your medical history. An endometrial biopsy can determine whether or not your symptoms point to endometrial cancer or some other cause.

Many symptoms of benign conditions, such as fibroids and polyps (uterine growths common in menopause), are similar to those of endometrial cancer. This "symptom mimic" makes it even more important that you report any change from what you consider normal for you to your doctor or health care provider.

One in fifty-seven women will develop ovarian cancer over the course of her life; it's the fourth leading cause of cancer deaths in women in the United States. Every year, U.S. doctors diagnose over 23,000 cases of this cancer, and more than 14,000 women die from it. Ovarian cancer occurs most often in women who are approaching the age of menopause. This cancer is a silent killer with symptoms that can be mild, vague, and similar to those of many other conditions and diseases. If detected early, while still in the ovary (called Stage I), this cancer is curable about 90 percent of the time. But if the cancer spreads to the pelvis or beyond (Stage III or IV), the five-year survival rate drops dramatically. Taking all stages into consideration, this cancer's overall five-year survival rate is somewhere around 40 percent.

Sadly, early ovarian cancer has few symptoms, so it makes sense to know your risk factors and your family history. Risk factors for ovarian cancer include:

- A family history of ovarian, breast, colon, rectal, endometrial, or pancreatic cancer increases a woman's risks considerably. The severity of increased risk is higher if there has been one of these cancers in a first-degree relative, such as a mother, sister, or daughter.
- A woman's risk of developing ovarian cancer also rises with the total number of times she has ovulated; again, exposure to estrogen has an impact on the woman's overall risks. In other words, not having

had any children or not taking the birth control pills at any point in your life means your ovaries have been working overtime, compared to women in the average population.

QUESTIONS?

What should I do if I think I might have ovarian cancer?
Contact your health care provider or see a gynecological oncologist. To learn more about this disease call the National Cancer Institute's Cancer Information Service (CIS) at ☎1-800-4-CANCER (☎1-800-422-6237) or visit its ovarian cancer information Web site at ✐*http://cancernet.nci.nih.gov/wyntk_pubs/ovarian.htm.*

Symptoms of ovarian cancer are vague, especially in the early stage, but can include pain, pressure, or swelling in your abdomen; gas, nausea, and indigestion; unexplained changes in your bowel movements; changes in your weight; fatigue; or pain during intercourse. If you exhibit any of these symptoms, talk to your doctor. He or she can perform a sonogram (ultrasound examination of the pelvis) to determine if your ovaries have any abnormalities. In addition, your health care provider may choose to obtain a blood test called CA-125 to check for a certain protein that can point to the presence of ovarian tumors. It is not a perfect test. An elevated result does not always mean ovarian cancer—it can point to liver problems, colon conditions such as diverticulitis, and other illnesses. Inaccurate results with this blood test (a false-positive) are highest in premenopausal women, so check with your doctor about the usefulness of taking the test and whether it's covered by your insurance. Of course, your health care provider physically palpates your ovaries every year during your pelvic examination to detect any changes in their size or shape. In most cases, a combination of symptoms and physical examination findings lead to a formal diagnostic series of tests for ovarian cancer. That's why now, more than ever, it's critical that you report any unusual physical symptoms or changes in your normal menstrual cycle to your health care provider.

Fibroids, Polyps, and Other Sources of Heavy or Irregular Bleeding

Irregular bleeding isn't uncommon during perimenopause. Because you ovulate less frequently during this time, your body's estrogen levels often are unchecked by progesterone. As a result, your uterine lining can develop abnormal cell changes that lead to unusually heavy bleeding or spotting.

As you've learned, irregular bleeding can have a number of causes, but two relatively common benign causes are fibroids and polyps. Fibroids are benign growths of muscle tissue that develop within the wall of the uterus, on the uterine lining, or on the outside of the uterus. Two out of five women in their forties can expect to develop these growths.

Fibroids within the uterine lining can cause abnormal bleeding because of the way they distort the lining and prevent it from shedding normally. Fibroids can sometimes become quite large. Their sheer size alone can cause problems, such as pelvic discomfort, bloating, or pain during intercourse. If you have unusually heavy or midcycle bleeding, your doctor probably will check for the presence of fibroids.

Fibroids usually shrink after menopause. As a result, your doctor may or may not choose to treat them with surgery or drugs, depending upon the severity of your symptoms. Conservative treatment options are now also available, usually done as out-patient surgery—a hysteroscopy. In this sophisticated dilation and curettage (D and C) procedure, a small (one-eighth-inch) camera lens and instrument port is inserted into the cervix to locate the polyps and remove all of them at that time. Although pain is usually minimal, you may request mild sedation during the procedure, and analgesics afterwards.

Polyps are smaller benign growths on the lining of the uterus. Science and medicine have yet to explain why polyps develop in some women, and not in others. Polyps bleed, just like fibroids, but because they typically are small, they're unlikely to cause the amount of blood loss associated with fibroids. When a health care provider diagnoses polyps (usually through an ultrasound test or a biopsy sample), he or she can remove them through a simple out-patient procedure in which the doctor snips the polyps from the uterine lining. This procedure usually involves a hysteroscopy, similar to that used to remove fibroids.

A common cause of abnormal bleeding is a precancerous condition of the lining of the uterus—endometrial hyperplasia. This excessive growth of the uterine lining can result from relatively low levels of progesterone. If diagnosed when still in its early stages, it can be treated medically. Untreated endometrial hyperplasia can develop into endometrial cancer.

FACTS

The least common cause of irregular bleeding is cancer. But, because endometrial cancer can masquerade as common irregular or heavy menstrual bleeding, it's important to talk to your doctor when your periods become too heavy, too frequent, or vary noticeably from your own personal norm.

Osteoporosis and Age

Osteoporosis—the loss of bone mass that results in porous, fragile bones—threatens nearly 28 million people in the United States, 80 percent of whom are women. According to the National Osteoporosis Foundation, 8 million women have osteoporosis and millions more have low bone density. Half of all women over the age of fifty will suffer an osteoporosis-related bone fracture at some time during their lives. Most of these fractures are preventable if a doctor diagnoses the early stages of osteoporosis, called osteopenia, at a time when preventable measures are possible.

Estrogen helps prevent the loss of bone density, and that's what makes osteoporosis such a growing threat for menopausal women. Hip fractures, crumbling vertebrae (the small bones that make up your spine), and the familiar stooped posture of many elderly women are just some of the all-too-common effects of this disease.

Bone loss begins early; by age thirty-five, your body begins to lose more bone material than it generates. Although at age thirty-five this decline is very gradual, the loss of bone material speeds up dramatically as estrogen levels drop off during perimenopause. In the five to seven years that follow menopause, the average woman can lose up to 20 percent of her bone mass, which usually signals the onset of osteoporosis.

The first outright symptom of osteoporosis may be a fractured hip or crumbled vertebrae that happens as the result of no more than a mild bump. Unfortunately, by the time such a break occurs, the disease has already done a lot of damage to your body's framework. Health care providers, therefore, depend on family medical history and sound prevention methods to stop osteoporosis before it strikes. Beyond age and the low estrogen levels that may be present in perimenopause, risk factors for osteoporosis include a family history of the disease; a small, thin frame; a diet low in calcium; or a history of eating disorders such as anorexia or bulimia (in which estrogen levels usually drop and menstrual periods often cease). Smoking, excessive use of alcohol, and a lack of exercise can contribute to osteoporosis, as well.

Some medications, such as corticosteroids, thyroid hormone replacement medications, and anticonvulsants, can contribute to bone loss. If your doctor prescribes these medications, be sure you have discussed your family health history and personal risks for osteoporosis.

By the time you've reached perimenopause, you've passed the age when you could continue to develop a stronger, healthier skeleton. Your goals now should be to slow calcium loss and maintain your bones' current strength. A healthy diet that's rich in calcium, plenty of weight-bearing exercise, and regular bone testing are just some of the ways you can maintain good bone health after menopause. (See Chapter 8 for more information on diagnosis, treatment, and prevention options.)

Urinary Tract Disorders and Yeast Infections

During perimenopause, about 40 percent of women experience some form of urogenital changes—changes to the vagina, genitals, and urinary tract. The most common of these changes result from vaginal atrophy, the thinning and drying of vaginal tissue that results from depleted estrogen levels. Thin, unelastic vaginal tissue is more easily irritated and broken, and therefore more prone to infections such as vaginitis, yeast infections, and urinary tract infections (UTIs). The severity of these disorders ranges from mildly irritating to very painful.

Most women have experienced some type of vaginitis (a swollen, red, irritated vaginal area) at some point in life. These infections include bacterial vaginosis, yeast infections, and trichomoniasis. During perimenopause, fluctuating hormone levels can contribute to the frequency and severity of these infections. Bacteria in the vagina, obesity, diabetes, and antibiotics are other contributors. The symptoms of these vaginal infections include burning and itching in the vaginal area and a discharge.

If you've had yeast infections before and are relatively certain that you're suffering from this type of infection, you can use any of the available over-the-counter creams and other treatments. But if you experience new or unusual symptoms, or the symptoms continue or recur (especially after using an over-the-counter medication), see your physician for a full diagnosis and treatment. And although you can't prevent all vaginal infections, here are some ways to try to avoid them:

- Don't wear tight clothes (such as jeans) that block air circulation to your lower body, and don't wear underpants to bed at night.
- Wear underwear and pantyhose with cotton crotches (avoid pantyhose if you can).
- Be clean, clean, clean; wash your genital area thoroughly, front to back, every day, but . . .
- Stay away from heavily perfumed and deodorizing soaps, douches, sprays, tampons, and pads, and use white unscented toilet paper. All of those perfumes and deodorant chemicals can dry out your skin and contribute to acid-level imbalances in your vagina that can lead to infections.

Fewer layers of clothing are better than too many (though layering the clothes on your upper body is a good idea when you suffer from hot flashes); looser is better than too tight; and natural fabrics such as cotton are better than spandex and other "unbreathable" blends. After exercising, swimming, or otherwise working up a sweat, change out of sweaty clothes and get into something clean and dry.

FACTS

If vaginal dryness is a problem for you, your doctor might reco-mmend more frequent sex as a treatment! Sexual arousal—even from masturbation—is a great way to help keep your vaginal tissues moist and flexible and stave off the effects of vaginal atrophy.

Urinary tract infections (UTIs) are common in women of all ages, but can be particularly persistent following menopause. In addition to the susceptibility of thin, dry vaginal tissue to infection, the lactobacilli organisms that help fight off bacterial infections in the vagina decline after menopause. And, as the bladder muscles weaken with age, the bladder doesn't empty completely, which can contribute to the buildup of bacteria. UTIs, including cystitis and urethritis, are caused by bacteria (usually from skin around the anus) traveling through the urethra and reaching the bladder, or even the kidneys. These bacteria trigger infections that result in symptoms such as pain or burning during urination; sudden, strong, and frequent urges to urinate; fever and chills; and even pain in your back, side, or abdomen.

The symptoms of more complicated UTIs may vary. If untreated, the bacteria from the bladder can rise to the kidneys. If you have painful urination, accompanied by pain in your back and fever, you may have a kidney infection. Kidney infections can result in chronic and even life-threatening consequences if untreated, so call your doctor immediately if you have these symptoms. If you have painful and quite frequent urination, you may have a bladder infection (sometimes called cystitis). Again, these infections can grow much worse if untreated, so you need to contact your doctor if you experience them. Sometimes more than one course of antibiotics or a different type of antibiotic is necessary to completely eradicate the bacteria.

If recurrent UTIs or symptoms that resemble UTIs become a problem for you, your doctor or health care provider might recommend estrogen cream or HRT to help rejuvenate your vaginal tissue. The estrogen helps increase the blood circulation to this area and restores natural secretions, thus making the entire vagina less susceptible to trauma. But you might be able to avoid some of these infections or discomforts through some simple, healthy habits:

- Wipe from front to back, so you don't push bacteria from your anus over your vaginal tissue.
- Drink lots of fluids (water is best) and urinate frequently to keep your urethra (the opening to the bladder) flushed out.
- Keep your vaginal area clean and chemical-free; wash your genital area daily and avoid any feminine hygiene products that contain additional chemicals, such as deodorant tampons, sanitary pads, and panty liners.
- Practice clean, safe sex, and always urinate after sex to flush bacteria from your urethra. It's a good idea for both partners to wash hands and genitals before having sex.
- Use a water-based lubricant (rather than an oil-based product such as petroleum jelly) to reduce friction during intercourse.

Assessing Your Health History

Everyone tells you that you inherited your father's temper and your mother's beautiful smile, but what else did your parents and grandparents hand down to you? Knowing your family's medical history is one of the best tools you have for predicting your future health. Many of the health risks that deserve your attention as you approach the age of menopause have risk factors associated with your personal health history and the health history of your immediate family. Your doctor or health care provider will want and need to know this information in order to monitor your health, prescribe appropriate treatment, and recommend appropriate preventative measures. Though this information is always important to your health care provider, it becomes essential as you enter perimenopause. If you have children, this information is important to them, as well.

Start Asking Questions

Most health care providers ask you to fill out a health history during your first appointment. If you aren't well versed in the medical history of your parents, grandparents, and siblings, talk to your family members ahead of time to gather this information. You'll want to gather medical information about as many of your family members as possible, but remember that your immediate family matters most. You can draw up your own form, fill it in for each family member, and take the forms with you to your medical appointment. For each family member, you should list the name, sex, relationship to you, year of birth, and year and cause of death. Then, note whether that person was ever diagnosed with any of the following health problems:

- ❏ heart disease
- ❏ high cholesterol
- ❏ coronary bypass surgery
- ❏ stroke
- ❏ breast cancer
- ❏ cervical cancer
- ❏ ovarian cancer
- ❏ other cancer (list)
- ❏ obesity
- ❏ allergies
- ❏ depression

- ❏ heart attack
- ❏ high blood pressure
- ❏ angina
- ❏ osteoporosis
- ❏ lung cancer
- ❏ endometrial cancer
- ❏ colon cancer
- ❏ diabetes
- ❏ emphysema
- ❏ alcoholism
- ❏ Alzheimer's

- ❏ schizophrenia or other psychiatric disorders (list)
- ❏ miscarriages, stillbirths, or other problems in pregnancy

If members of your immediate family died at an early age from medical conditions (not accidental deaths), you should also ask other family members about those individuals' lifestyles and living conditions. Did they smoke or drink excessively? Did their jobs or living environment expose them to potentially toxic substances? Did they seem to be under a great deal of stress, or were there any other factors that might have contributed to an early death? The more you—and your doctor—know about the health problems that your relatives have experienced, the better able you'll be to develop a lifestyle and health maintenance plan to help protect you from inherited risks.

FACTS

If any member of your immediate family has been diagnosed with cancer, you need to add some important information to that person's medical history. At what age was the person's cancer diagnosed? What was his or her treatment history? Did the cancer recur? This type of information can indicate whether the cancer was genetically transmitted.

Don't Forget Your Own History

Your doctor or health care professional will want to know the same information about you that you've gathered about your family members. Your medical history form (most health care providers will ask you to fill one of these forms out) will also ask about what illnesses, diseases, surgeries, hospitalizations, and other health issues you've experienced. Gather the information before your doctor's appointment, so you're fully prepared to discuss your history. Try to remember (or better yet, write down) dates of surgeries and hospitalizations. If you've taken birth control pills prescribed by another doctor, write down the brand name and the dates during which you took them. And don't forget your menstrual calendar (see Chapter 3).

Your After-Forty Health Maintenance Plan

Okay, you've reviewed some of the health issues that you need to keep in mind after age forty, and know how to put together your family and personal health histories. All of this information lays the foundation for building a strong, effective health plan that will help you and your health care provider keep tabs on your health in the years ahead. Some common sense lifestyle guidelines and regular medical examinations are your ticket to a happy, healthy (and youthful) middle age.

Your Contributions to Your Health

Medical science can't do it all. You have to take responsibility for the most important part of your health maintenance—healthy living. Some components of a savvy, postforty health life plan go without saying; but let's list them, anyway:

- Eat a varied diet that's high in vegetables, fruit, complex carbohydrates, and plenty of calcium, vitamins, and minerals (see Chapter 13).
- Drink lots of water—at least one quart—every day.
- Exercise regularly—thirty minutes a day, four or more days a week is a minimum recommendation, but every day is better, and any exercise is better than none. Include both weight-bearing and aerobic exercise in your plan (see Chapter 14).
- Stop smoking. Stop smoking. Stop smoking.
- Relax. Stress and fatigue contribute to a wide variety of illnesses and diseases, in ways that we probably don't even fully comprehend. A calm, rested body and mind are your best defense against illness and disease.
- If you're sexually active, have your partner use a condom and continue using contraception. Remember, until you've been diagnosed as having gone through menopause (by either an FSH test or after having passed an entire year without a menstrual period), you are still fertile and can still get pregnant.
- Give yourself regular, monthly breast exams.
- Get regular, annual checkups, including any special tests for your risks.

Breast self-exams are your first line of defense against breast cancer. Ask your health care provider to demonstrate how to check your breasts for lumps or growths or visit ✐*www.cancer.org* for a good, visual guide to this procedure. Self-exams must be accompanied by annual mammograms after age forty, especially when you have a positive family history.

Your Annual Checkups

Your doctor or health care provider will discuss the type of tests that you should undergo every year, based on your family and personal medical histories and your lifestyle. Listed below are some of the components that any annual exam should include:

WHAT?	WHO?	HOW OFTEN?
Pap smear	Every woman	Every year
Pelvic and rectal exam	Every woman	Every year
Breast exam	Every woman	Every year by a professional health care provider; every month by you
Blood pressure	Every woman	Every year
Cholesterol	Every woman	Every three years if initial test is normal; more often as prescribed
Mammogram	Every woman age forty+	Baseline at forty; every one to two years to age fifty; then every year
Fecal occult blood test	Every woman	Annually after age fifty; after age forty if you have a family history
Electrocardiogram (ECG)	Anyone with two risk factors (family history, heart disease, high cholesterol, smoking, diabetes, high blood pressure)	Every three to five years

WHAT?	WHO?	HOW OFTEN?
Bone density	Any woman with risk factors for osteoporosis, every woman age sixty-five and older	Every year
Sigmoidoscopy	Every woman age fifty+	Every three to five years
Skin cancer check	Every woman	Annually by professional, monthly by you
Blood glucose check	Every woman age forty-five+	Every three years

These will help you stay on top of your changing body as it approaches and moves through menopause.

CHAPTER 7

Menopause and Heart Disease

Though it's the number one killer of American women today, few women would name heart disease as a major health concern. The problems that contribute to heart disease can grow silently over a number of years. Even the first signs of serious heart illness, such as a heart attack or stroke, can be attributed to other causes and therefore go unrecognized.

What Is Heart Disease?

The term heart disease refers to any disorder or condition of the heart and blood vessels; these diseases fall under the catchall category of cardiovascular disease. Coronary artery disease is a common form of heart disease that occurs when arteries become lined with heavy deposits of plaque—a substance made up of fat, calcium, and other minerals. The plaque buildup narrows the diameter of the vessels, thus limiting the amount of blood that can flow through the arteries, contributing to a condition known as atherosclerosis. Blood carries oxygen to all of the body's muscles, including the heart. As plaque narrows or blocks the coronary arteries, the heart is starved of oxygen, which can lead to a heart attack—and damage the heart muscle itself.

FACTS

Atherosclerosis can also contribute to the plaque buildup in the carotid arteries that carry oxygen-rich blood to the brain. The plaque buildup can lead to the formation of blood clots, which can break loose from the inside of the vessel walls and be carried to your brain, causing a *stroke*. In 1998, stroke killed twice as many American women as were killed by breast cancer.

Other heart diseases include congestive heart failure, diseases of the heart valves, irregular heartbeats (arrhythmias), and congenital heart diseases. But for women entering menopause, the threat of heart disease comes mainly from coronary artery disease, the atherosclerosis that contributes to it, and the heart attacks and stroke that all of these conditions can lead to.

The Symptoms of Heart Disease

Unfortunately, coronary artery disease can reach an advanced state without ever issuing a warning sign or symptom. The first major symptom you're likely to experience is a chest pain called angina—a squeezing, heaviness, or tightness in your chest that happens when your heart is starved of oxygen. You might feel this pain when you're exercising, climbing stairs, or rushing to a meeting, or when you're feeling stressed out or highly emotional. At first, the feeling may be just a momentary pressure that passes quickly if you stop and rest for a moment. However, as the arteries become narrower, you're likely to feel the pain again, and it may radiate down your left arm and shoulder, up through your neck and jaw, or down your back. As the atherosclerosis progresses, the pain of angina can become worse. Angina is your warning that you have heart disease and are at risk for suffering a heart attack.

On the other hand, you may have no warning at all. Many people are unaware that they suffer from any kind of heart disease until they have a heart attack, but women are more likely than men to experience the warning pangs of angina before a full heart attack occurs. Because the symptoms of angina are very much like those of a heart attack, it's critical that you report those symptoms to your health care provider immediately for diagnosis.

According to the American Medical Association, as many as one-third of heart attacks go undiagnosed in women—or are attributed to some other cause, such as indigestion. If you have any of the symptoms of a heart attack, contact your doctor immediately.

When a Heart Attack Hits

If one or more of your coronary arteries become completely blocked, you can have a heart attack. Over 200,000 women die of heart attack every year in this country, and many thousand more suffer an attack and survive. A heart attack can be mild, moderate, or severe, depending upon the amount of damage to the heart muscle. If only a small area of the heart is deprived of blood, the healthy heart tissue surrounding it continues to work, allowing the damaged part of the heart to heal as new vessels grow in from the healthy areas. But if damage occurs in several of these small areas, they can combine to damage the heart beyond repair.

The symptoms of heart attack vary; in some cases, the attack is so minor that no noticeable symptoms occur. In fact, many heart attacks in women are misdiagnosed as indigestion. But in many other cases, the symptoms of heart attack are evident; we just need to recognize them. Those symptoms include:

- A crushing or dull pain in the chest
- Pain in the left shoulder, arm, neck, or back
- Sweating, nausea, shortness of breath
- Fatigue or dizziness
- Burning pain in the midchest area similar to heartburn or indigestion

FACTS

Heart attacks affect different women in different ways. If you have more than one heart attack, your second one may feel different from the first. That's why it's important that you watch for all signs of heart attack—don't be too quick to dismiss any of them as normal aches and pains.

Only rarely do heart attacks cause the heart to stop functioning completely. More often, you have a chance to make a big difference in the amount of damage your heart receives and your chances for a recovery. But you must act quickly; most heart attack damage occurs within the first two hours after you feel the pain. If you have any reason to suspect you may be having an attack—a personal history of angina or a family history of heart disease—be prepared to get help. Sit or lie down for a minute or two. If you continue to feel the symptoms, call an ambulance or 911 and tell the operator you might be having a heart attack. Then, follow that operator's instructions until the ambulance arrives. For example, the operator is likely to ask you to take an aspirin as you wait for the paramedics.

If you have the symptoms of heart attack, don't drive yourself to the hospital and don't avoid calling for help because you aren't certain the pains you feel are a heart attack. You're in no position to diagnose your symptoms, and no one expects you to. If there was ever a situation where the old "better safe than sorry" expression applies, this is it. Be smart. Get medical attention immediately.

Women, Menopause, and Heart Disease

Now that you know what heart disease is, you might be wondering why you need to be concerned about it now. After all, if you're just entering perimenopause, you're probably in your forties, or if you've just experienced menopause, you might be in your early fifties. You're far from some old-timer who needs to worry about a failing heart—right?

Actually, you're right about the first part of that statement, but wrong about the last. At forty or fifty, you're far from being an old-timer, but heart disease doesn't strike only the elderly. Heart disease is the number one killer of women age fifty and over. One in five women has some type of heart or blood vessel disease, and every year nearly half a million women in the United States die from cardiovascular diseases.

Between 1988 and 1998, death rates from coronary heart disease in women declined by approximately 25 percent, and death rates from all cardiovascular diseases in women declined by nearly 19 percent. These drops are probably due to increased awareness of heart disease incidence in women and earlier diagnosis through cholesterol screening.

Women in their childbearing years are statistically less prone to heart disease than are men of the same age. According to the American Heart Association, "Menopause itself appears to increase a woman's risks of coronary heart disease and stroke." Your risk of heart disease increases when you reach menopause—then just keeps on increasing. If your menopause occurs naturally, the risk rises slowly. But if menopause results from surgery, the risks can rise dramatically and quickly.

What's Menopause Got to Do with It?

If women have less risk of heart disease before menopause than do men of the same age, with the same contributing risk factors, why does their postmenopausal risk surpass that of men? To understand this surge in risk, it's important to understand some of the root causes of heart disease in any individual. Though later sections of this chapter discuss these risk factors in detail, one of the most important contributors to heart disease is high blood cholesterol levels. When you develop high blood cholesterol levels, you have too much artery-clogging fat in your bloodstream. The diminished supply of estrogen that occurs with menopause, weight gain, and the aging of your cardiovascular system all contribute to developing high cholesterol levels.

Do ERT and HRT Lower Your Risk?

A number of medical researchers and scientists believe that a woman's own natural estrogen might help protect her from heart disease, but they're still studying how the hormone may have that effect. Estrogen plays an important role in maintaining healthy, strong muscle tissue, including the muscle of the heart. Estrogen also has an impact on the blood's level of triglycerides and low-density lipoproteins (LDL) or "bad" cholesterol, both of which can contribute to atherosclerosis and heart attack. Some studies have shown that estrogen contributes to healthy, reactive arteries and an increased blood flow. As a result, blood vessels are better able to relax and respond to exercise and physical stress by dilating and providing more blood flow when needed.

Does that mean that you can avoid heart disease through estrogen replacement or hormone replacement therapies? Not necessarily. According to the American Heart Association (AHA), estrogen replacement therapy (ERT) does have a positive effect on several risk factors for heart disease and stroke. For example, oral forms of both ERT and HRT increase the level of HDL cholesterol and lower the level of LDL cholesterol. Estrogen administered in the form of a skin patch also has some beneficial effects on your lipid profile, although it may take longer for these benefits to show up on your blood tests. Even so, the AHA doesn't recommend that you use either of these therapies as a replacement for cholesterol-lowering drugs if you're battling high blood cholesterol levels.

One twenty-five-year-long study, known as the Harvard Nurses' Health Study, linked ERT and HRT with a lower risk of death from heart disease—a benefit that lasted even after ten years of hormone treatment. Another study, the Heart and Estrogen-Progestin Replacement Study (HERS), focused on postmenopausal women who already had coronary heart disease. After approximately four years of follow-up, that study indicated that HRT did not reduce the participants' overall risk of heart attack or death from coronary heart disease as much as previously expected, nor did it have any major impact on their overall risk of stroke. Partial results of a new, ongoing study funded by the NIH actually found a small but increased risk of nonfatal heart attack, stroke, deep vein blood clot, and pulmonary embolus in women taking one form of HRT for several years. There has been no increased risk in women taking estrogen alone so far

FACTS

The American Heart Association's complete recommendations for women considering using HRT or ERT to combat heart disease— "Women and Cardiovascular Diseases"—is available on the AHA's Web site at *www.americanheart.org*. To contact the AHA, call 1-800-242-8721.

Studies continue and you can expect new developments in our understanding of the role of estrogen, estrogen replacement, and heart disease in women. Medical experts continue to try to assimilate the results of numerous studies, but this process can be difficult due to differences in the populations of women who entered the studies and the studies' criteria. For now, you need to weigh the potential benefits and risks of any treatment for heart disease, and discuss them carefully with your health care provider. (See Chapter 11.)

Heart Disease Risk Factors

As with most killers, heart disease is rarely the product of a single event or condition. Heart disease has long been the focus of intense medical study, contributing to the knowledge about the many illnesses and conditions that can contribute to its development. Some risk factors are yours for life—risks associated with your age, sex, race, and genetic inheritance—so you have to construct your healthy life plan with the idea that those risks will always be present. Fortunately, the majority of factors that promote heart disease are controllable. The following sections take a closer look at all of these risk factors—whether they're the products of fate or folly.

The Risk Factors You Own

The key risk factors for developing heart disease that cannot be controlled are few. Women face two unchangeable risks for developing heart disease:

Growing older: The older you get, the greater your risk for developing heart disease. Four out of five people who die of it are sixty-five or older. And the older women are when they suffer a heart attack, the more likely they are to die of it.

Heredity: If your parents had heart disease, you're more likely to develop it. Sometimes it is because of a propensity to high cholesterol levels. Race-associated conditions can have an impact on heart disease risk, as well. Because African Americans can have more severe high blood pressure, they have an elevated risk for developing coronary heart disease. Mexican Americans, Native Americans, Asian Americans, and native Hawaiians also have a higher risk for developing the disease.

Having these unchangeable risk factors doesn't mean you're destined to suffer from heart disease. But it does mean that you need to be extra vigilant about controlling the risks you can change.

High Cholesterol

High blood cholesterol is a major risk factor for developing heart disease. After menopause, women tend to develop high levels of triglycerides (a form of fat), in addition to high levels of low-density lipoprotein (LDL), cholesterol. At the same time, their levels of high-density lipoprotein (HDL) can diminish. All of these factors lead to out-of-balance blood cholesterol levels, too much fat in the bloodstream, and the buildup of artery-clogging plaque in the pathways that channel oxygen rich blood to the heart and brain. For every 1 percent reduction in elevated blood cholesterol levels, you get a 2 to 3 percent reduction in your chances of having a heart attack.

Don't misunderstand the issue about cholesterol; cholesterol is a natural, essential substance in the bloodstream. The fraction of your total cholesterol that is HDL cholesterol is actually a protein that helps keep all fats and cholesterols moving through your bloodstream (and not glued to your arterial walls), so it actually helps you stave off a potential heart attack. LDL cholesterol moves cholesterol through the rest of your body—but it also has a tendency to linger in your arteries and stick to the walls. Elevated levels of triglycerides may or may not indicate that you're headed for a heart attack, but as another type of fat in the bloodstream, their levels need to be monitored.

So how much is too much (or not enough) of these substances? While your total blood cholesterol level should remain below 200 mg/dl (milligrams per deciliter of blood), and anything over 239 mg/dl needs to be considered a high risk, here's how the individual cholesterol numbers should stack up:

- **HDL**—more than 60 mg/dl is a good number here, less than 35 mg/dl puts you at high risk.
- **LDL**—less than 130 mg/dl is desirable, up to 159 mg/dl is considered borderline high, and 160 mg/dl and higher is high risk.
- **Triglycerides**—less than 200 mg/dl is considered normal, up to 400 mg/dl is borderline high, 400 to 1,000 mg/dl is high, and over 1,000 mg/dl is way too high.

Though some research has indicated that high cholesterol levels in some people might be a result of heredity, a low-fat diet and regular exercise can help most people maintain healthy blood cholesterol levels. Where those efforts fall short, a variety of cholesterol-lowering drugs, called statins, have entered the market over the past several years. Recent studies have shown that these drugs do actually reduce your risk of dying from a heart disease. Although some of these drugs may have side effects, the medications currently on the market are considered safe and effective. Consult your physician; do not rely on a homeopath or other alternative health care if your lipid profile is abnormal.

FACTS

Triglycerides are a type of fat found in the blood, but more appealing types of this fat include butter, margarine, and vegetable oil. Eating these fats doesn't automatically result in high triglyceride blood levels, though; the partners in crime here seem to be overindulging in alcohol, being overweight, or having diabetes.

The effectiveness of HRT and ERT in managing blood cholesterol is still the subject of much medical research. Estrogen has been shown to reduce total blood cholesterol levels and to raise levels of HDL. But, recent studies indicate that some types of estrogen may actually slightly increase levels of triglycerides in the bloodstream. Your triglycerides may decrease if the estrogen in your prescription regimen is combined with just the right progestin for HRT. Though the AHA doesn't recommend ERT or HRT as a first defense against high cholesterol, you should discuss this option with your health care provider, who can make recommendations based on your complete health profile, family medical history, and current symptoms.

High Blood Pressure

High blood pressure (hypertension) is another silent plague of women age fifty-five and over. More than half of all women in that age group have blood pressure greater than 140/90 (the high-blood-pressure threshold), but few of them feel its effects. In fact, though some estimates say that one in four people in the United States suffers from high blood pressure, nearly one-third of those individuals are unaware of their condition. Even if you have had normal blood pressure all of your life, you might develop high blood pressure after menopause. And having high blood pressure makes you a prime candidate for developing heart disease. High blood pressure also contributes to kidney disease and can lead to congestive heart failure, heart attack, and stroke.

Like cholesterol, everyone needs blood pressure. After all, blood pressure results from the force of your heart pumping your blood through your veins. If you exercise or become excited, your heart rate increases, sending more blood through your system. If your arteries are clean and wide open, the blood flows freely; if they're narrow or blocked, the buildup of blood trying to course through your veins puts pressure on the arterial walls—and that's high blood pressure. If your arteries are clean and healthy, your blood pressure rises for a short period of time, then returns to normal as the blood moves through your circulatory system. If you have hypertension, however, your blood pressure is greater than 140/90, even when you're at rest; the extra pressure on your heart and arteries never lets up. If high blood pressure occurs in a person with atherosclerosis, the walls of the vessels are toughened and less elastic, and even less able to cope with stress.

FACTS

High blood pressure is a particular threat to African Americans, women over age thirty-five, heavy drinkers, obese women, and those with diabetes or kidney disease. However, a family history of high blood pressure isn't a strong risk indicator—one inheritance you can be happy to pass up.

Most doctors consider 120/80 the ideal blood pressure reading. Though some people have suffered from low blood pressure, it's a relatively uncommon occurrence and not life threatening. Regular exercise and a diet high in vegetables and fruit, but low in sodium, can help control high blood pressure. If diet, exercise, and weight loss (when indicated) don't bring blood pressure down, your health care provider may prescribe drug therapy.

Diabetes

Diabetes is another heart disease risk factor that is of particular concern to women. Nearly 6 million women in the United States have been diagnosed with diabetes, and another 2.5 million women have undiagnosed diabetes. Women who have diabetes are at a significantly greater risk of developing heart disease than their nondiabetic "sisters." Having diabetes ups your risk of heart disease and stroke by two to four times. Every year, over 60,000 Americans die of complications of diabetes, and the disease can lead to a host of other conditions, including kidney failure, blindness, and nerve disease.

Diabetes mellitus occurs when the body is unable to produce adequate amounts of insulin or efficiently use the insulin it produces (insulin resistance). Insulin is produced in the pancreas, and the body uses it to process the sugar and carbohydrates you consume into energy. Type 2 or adult onset diabetes is the most common form of the disease, and it usually occurs at middle age. Symptoms of diabetes include weight loss, blurred vision, intense thirst, fatigue, excessive urination, and hunger. Doctors test for diabetes through assessing the level of glucose (sugar) in your blood. If a random (nonfasting) glucose screening test is borderline or abnormal, or if your family history is very strong, the doctor may decide to repeat the test. In that test, the doctor may ask you to fast before the first blood sample is taken; then, after you drink a specifically prepared glucose solution, blood samples are taken again at two one-hour intervals. If two of the samples show an elevated blood sugar level, you're considered to be diabetic.

ESSENTIALS

The American Diabetes Association recommends that you have a fasting blood glucose test at age forty-five and every three years thereafter. For more information about diabetes, visit the ADA's Web site at *www.diabetes.org*, or call 800-342-2383.

Doctors don't know what causes the development of diabetes, and no drug can cure it. However, diabetes can be controlled—and sometimes disappears altogether—through diet, exercise, and weight loss. Statistics show that 80 to 90 percent of people with diabetes are overweight, and many have high blood pressure and/or lead inactive lives. Though a large number of diabetics require insulin or drug therapy, many others are able to control their disease through behavior modification, such as diet, exercise, and weight loss—a lifelong change that offers big rewards.

Obesity

Few diseases are as common and as potentially damaging (both emotionally and physically) as obesity. In fact, obesity has never been more common; the numbers of obese people in the United States continue to rise at alarming levels. The percentage of overweight Americans has risen by over 60 percent in the past decade, and nearly half of all American women are overweight or obese—conditions defined in general by a body weight more than 30 percent over the ideal for the body's height and frame, or having an abnormally high body mass index (BMI). Obesity is damaging in ways few nonobese people can imagine; unlike most other diseases, obesity is commonly viewed as a disease of weakness, self-indulgence, and laziness. Obese people often are the object of ridicule and disdain. Unlike other heart disease risk factors, obesity is plainly visible.

FACTS

The link between hypertension and obesity is particularly strong. The American Heart Association estimates that over 75 percent of all diagnosed hypertension is directly related to obesity.

Though obesity can result in obvious emotional distress, its health-damaging effects are even more insidious. Obesity is strongly linked to heart disease in ways that are still under study, but some research indicates that nearly 70 percent of diagnosed cases of heart disease may be directly linked to obesity. And obesity is a gateway disease for numerous other conditions, including diabetes, high blood pressure, high blood cholesterol levels, kidney disease, sleep apnea, depression, menstrual irregularities, joint disease, and even some forms of cancer.

Though weight gain in middle age isn't uncommon for both men and women, women are at special risk for heart disease from their postmenopausal weight gain. The reason is the location of the added weight; many women tend to add weight in their abdomen and upper body during menopause. This type of fat seems to be linked very closely with a number of other risk factors for heart disease, including diabetes. And at middle-age, women are particularly susceptible to weight gain. The body's metabolism begins to slow down during perimenopause; as a result, the body burns fewer calories, even at rest. So if a middle-aged woman continues to consume the same number of calories she consumed in her youth, chances are good that she will gain weight.

SSENTIALS Body mass index (BMI) is used to calculate both overweight and obesity, while height and weight tables offer another option for determining obesity. For more information about obesity and weight control, visit the National Institute of Diabetes and Digestive and Kidney Diseases at ✐*www.niddk.nih.gov.*

Though so many Americans suffer from obesity, researchers are still trying to determine all of the factors that contribute to it. Some contributors are controllable—things such as leading a sedentary lifestyle and consuming a high-fat, high-calorie diet. But if those factors were the only causes of obesity, fewer individuals would suffer from the disease. In fact, our sex, age, individual biological and genetic makeup, psychological condition, and environment each appear capable of playing a major role in the development of obesity.

Still, behavior modification is a powerful weapon against obesity. A low-calorie, low-fat, high-fiber diet and regular exercise are the first line of defense against this disease. But for many people, other methods prove helpful, including drug therapy, psychotherapy, hypnosis, acupuncture, and even surgery. As this disease continues to become more prevalent in our society, look for further discoveries and advancement in its treatment.

Smoking

Smoking tobacco is hard on your entire body, but it delivers a particularly hard blow to your heart. Each time you draw in a lungful of tobacco smoke, you temporarily increase your heart rate and blood pressure and deplete the oxygen in your bloodstream that should be going to feed your heart and other body tissues. If you smoke even one to four cigarettes a day, you're doubling your chances of having a heart attack—and very few smokers smoke four or fewer cigarettes in the average day. Smoke a pack or more, and your risk goes up four times. Over 30 percent of all deaths due to coronary heart disease are attributable to smoking. There's little disagreement in the health care profession about the dangers of tobacco addiction. Smoking is linked to innumerable other diseases and conditions, including a wide range of cardiovascular and other heart diseases, chronic lung diseases, and many forms of cancer. Smoking kills over 430,000 people in the United States each year.

But hey—you knew all of that, didn't you? And, you undoubtedly know that smoking-related diseases are incredibly preventable. Not only do even long-time smokers experience very immediate benefits from quitting, but also smokers who have already developed tobacco smoking-related diseases can benefit from kicking the habit. Your body begins repairing smoke-related damage within an hour after your last cigarette. Although all the studies haven't included women, some have shown that men who quit smoking can have the same risk of heart disease as nonsmokers within three to five years of quitting. If you're a smoker, the best thing you can do for your heart (and the rest of your body for that matter) is to stop smoking now.

FACTS

In 1999, the *New England Journal of Medicine* reported a study that found that nonsmokers exposed to environmental smoke have a higher risk of coronary heart disease than those who aren't. So don't be shy—ask smokers to smoke outside.

Smoking is an incredibly addictive habit, however, that hooks users physically, psychologically, and emotionally. If you can't just throw down the pack and stop smoking, you're in the majority; talk to your doctor or health care provider about smoking cessation programs, nicotine replacement therapy, and other techniques that can help you kick the habit. If you have children, remind yourself of how important you are to them as a role model; your quitting smoking may help them decide not to start.

Controlling Your Risks

As you've probably determined by reading the previous sections on individual risk factors for developing heart disease, you actually can exercise (get it?) a great deal of control over your personal susceptibility to this disease and the conditions that contribute to it. Though you might have a genetic susceptibility to high blood pressure, high cholesterol, or diabetes, or your age itself may increase your chances of contracting heart disease, you can take positive action to manage your overall risks. Here are some suggestions:

- **Eat a low-fat, low-cholesterol, high-fiber diet.** The less saturated fat you consume, the better you'll be able to manage blood cholesterol levels. Try to build your diet around fresh fruits, vegetables, and whole grains. Limit the amount of animal fat, meat, and dairy products you consume, and go easy on the salt—especially if you suffer from high blood pressure. And eat some soy; eating 25 grams of soy protein—from soy milk, veggie burgers, or tofu—a day can help lower your LDL cholesterol level by as much as 5 to 10 percent. (For more information about the benefits and sources of soy, see Chapter 13.)
- **Manage your weight.** Ask your health care provider to help you determine what your weight should be and how you can best reach and maintain that weight. The first step to weight management is diet management. Eat a low-calorie, low-fat diet, and weigh yourself regularly. To track the kinds and amounts of foods you eat, keep a

food diary of your meals, including calorie and fat gram count. No matter what other lifestyle changes you make, being overweight or obese can dramatically increase your risks of suffering from some form of heart disease.

- **Exercise regularly.** Physical activity not only helps control obesity, but also helps dramatically reduce the severity of many conditions that contribute to heart disease. And the really good news about exercise is that you can get it just about any way you like. Walking, vacuuming the floor, taking stairs instead of elevators, and dancing are all great ways to up your activity level. The Surgeon General recommends thirty minutes of exercise, at least three days a week, but an hour of exercise, four days a week is better. Your exercise should boost your heart rate, but it doesn't have to be a "killer" routine. Try to combine both weight training (such as lifting weights) and aerobic (swimming, walking, running) exercises, preceded and followed by a series of stretching movements in your routine.

- **Drink alcohol in moderation.** If you drink alcohol, keep your consumption to no more than one drink a day.

- **Stop smoking.** Now—use whatever means necessary.

- **Find ways to avoid or relieve stress.** Being stressed out is not only unpleasant but also hard on your heart. When you're under stress, your heart rate can go up, your breathing can become shallow, and all of your muscles can become tense. If you want your heart and brain to be nourished by a strong, healthy flow of oxygenated blood, learn to keep stress to a minimum. Exercise helps, as does relaxation therapy, meditation, and quiet time spent enjoying the things you love.

CHAPTER 8

Maintaining Bone Health

Osteoporosis is a threat every woman should take seriously, and that threat grows even more serious as menopause approaches. Your best defense against osteoporosis is to understand your risks for developing this disease and to follow a sensible plan for minimizing those risks and protecting your bones—for the rest of your life.

Close-up on Osteoporosis

Osteoporosis is a degenerative bone disease that every woman should view as a potential enemy. According to the National Osteoporosis Foundation, of the more than 28 million people in the United States threatened by this disease, 10 million men and women already have osteoporosis; the other 18 million individuals have low bone mass that places them at an increased risk of progressing to osteoporosis. What is really frightening: 80 percent of the 28 million Americans either diagnosed or at heightened risk are women.

If your first instinct upon reading these statistics is to dash out and stock up on calcium supplements, hold on a minute. Your best weapon against osteoporosis is knowledge; take a moment to get the facts on this disease. Then, you can get the calcium supplements—and follow the simple prescription for bone health offered later in this chapter.

FACTS

Fifty percent of women with osteoporosis don't have any recognizable risk factors, so all women should take precautions; eat a healthy, calcium-rich diet; get plenty of weight-bearing exercise; and have regular bone density testing.

What Is Osteoporosis?

Osteoporosis is a disease in which your bones lose density. When you have osteoporosis, your bone tissue deteriorates, leaving your bones structurally weak and susceptible to fractures. Typically, victims of osteoporosis suffer fractures in their hips, spinal vertebrae, and wrists, but any bone in the body can crumble when this disease progresses to an advanced state.

Many people think of their adult bones the same way they view their home's 2 x 4 framework: a stable and unchanging support for the growing, vital parts of the body's makeup. But bones are alive. Bone tissue is in a constant state of evolution, as the body replaces old bone cells with new bone cells. When you're a child, your bones have a lot of growing to do, so your body produces much more new bone than it takes back in through resorption (the process of absorbing old bone cells back into the body).

But around age thirty, your body reaches a stage of peak bone mass, where your bones are as large and dense as they will ever be. At that stage, resorption slowly begins to outpace bone production. If resorption becomes too rapid or if bone cell production becomes too slow, you're at risk for developing osteoporosis. If you didn't build your bones to their optimum size during the years leading to peak bone mass, your risk is even greater.

Young girls need to build bone density, but it's not a subject that interests most teenagers. So, if you have a young daughter or niece, make sure she's taking in adequate amounts of calcium, especially during her early teen years' growth spurt.

Right now, there is no cure for osteoporosis. But you can slow the progress of the disease dramatically through a treatment plan involving some combination of medication, diet, and exercise. Recent experiments with drugs that may actually help rebuild lost bone tissue offer true encouragement to victims of this disease and those who treat them. But remember, prevention is easier than treatment.

How Osteoporosis Strikes

Osteoporosis, even today, is underdiagnosed and undertreated. Like many deadly diseases, osteoporosis gains much of its power through its ability to progress silently without any readily apparent signs or symptoms. Bone tissue loss isn't painful in its early stages—everyone experiences it every day. Weak bones don't ache, or creak, or exhibit any other kind of warning. In fact, osteoporosis frequently is diagnosed only after someone suffers a bone fracture. And even then, if the person who suffered the break and/or her doctor doesn't suspect that the break could be related to osteoporosis, and follow up with the proper diagnostic tests, the disease can remain undiagnosed and untreated.

Osteoporotic bones lose mass very slowly; over time, the bones become so fragile that they can break under very slight strain. Every year, osteoporosis is responsible for:

- 300,000 hip fractures
- 700,000 vertebral fractures
- 250,000 wrist fractures
- 300,000 fractures at other sites

Some of these figures may be underestimates, since certain fractures aren't even recognized when they occur. The pain resulting from crumbled vertebrae might seem like a back strain, for example. If the broken bone goes unnoticed or, the break is apparent but no one connects it to the disease, osteoporosis continues to erode the bones until another fracture occurs. By the time the warning flag goes up, the disease may have advanced to a critical stage.

SSENTIALS

Ninety percent of all hip fractures are associated with osteoporosis and result from a fall. Most falls happen to women in their homes in the afternoon. When your legs lose strength, your eyesight becomes weaker (especially your peripheral vision), and your balance and flexibility diminish, you're more likely to fall and be unable to catch yourself. These changes can begin in your forties and fifties, making osteoporosis a real concern to you now.

Diagnosing the Disease

Because osteoporosis is such a well-hidden disease, your health care provider will turn to your health history (and your family's health history) to determine what your risk factors are for developing the disease. A close review of your osteoporosis risk profile will tell your health care provider how soon (and often) you need to be checked for the development of the disease.

The most common and effective diagnostic tool for osteoporosis is a bone density measurement known as a bone mineral density (BMD) test. BMD tests can measure the density of the bones in your spine, wrist, heel, and/or hip.

Fractures from minor accidents can indicate bone loss. If you have suffered a fracture after a minor fall, you should ask your doctor about conducting a BMD test. Other late signs of osteoporosis occur in many women age sixty-five and older, including stooped shoulders or a loss of height.

The most common type of bone density test is a dual energy X-ray absorptiometry (DXA) test. In this test, low-dose X-ray beams scan your lower (lumbar) spine and/or hips for ten to twenty minutes. The test isn't painful, and you're exposed to minimal radiation, so it's a safe and effective diagnostic tool. Other types of bone density scans use ultrasound to measure the bone mass in your heel or wrist, but aren't as conclusive as the DXA test. However, a quick office scan of the density of your heel or wrist still provides very useful knowledge, especially if you are relatively young (less than forty-five years old), and have risk factors for this condition. This type of peripheral bone density testing is a great screening tool, because it takes less than two minutes to perform, and most doctors can conduct the test right in the office during a routine visit.

Besides warning you about osteoporosis before you suffer a fracture, bone density tests can help you determine your rate of bone loss and help you gauge the effectiveness of your efforts to slow that loss. A BMD test can tell you how your bone density compares to that of healthy bone tissue from a person of your age and—more importantly—to that of an average twenty-five-year-old.

Menopause and Osteoporosis

As you've learned, women make up the vast majority of those diagnosed with osteoporosis. As you approach menopause, your chances for developing this disease increase dramatically. Here's why. Your bones are in a constant state of remodeling its bone tissue, by removing old bone tissue cells through resorption and creating new ones. But, as with many remodelers, the body is more adept at tearing down the old than at building the new. Your body depends upon its growth hormones—especially estrogen—to help pace the remodeling process.

Estrogen Loss Depletes Bone Tissue

So what role does estrogen play in this whole remodeling process? Estrogen protects your bones by controlling the amount of bone removed by resorption. When your estrogen levels drop after menopause (either gradually through natural menopause or dramatically as a result of induced menopause), your bones lose that protection. As a result, in the five to eight years following menopause, your bone loss can increase dramatically as your body adjusts to the loss of ovarian estrogen.

If you've gone through an early menopause, your body has endured a greater-than-normal estrogen loss and your risk of experiencing accelerated bone loss increases. And if you've ever experienced extensive or frequent bouts of amenorrhea (lack of periods), your bones have been through periods of accelerated bone loss due to a loss of estrogen protection.

FACTS

Your parathyroid gland secretes a hormone that controls the amount of calcium released by your bones into the bloodstream. If this gland becomes overactive (hyperparathyroidism), your bones can release too much calcium and contribute to the development of osteoporosis. This condition is particularly dangerous for women in menopause. The good news is that hyperparathyroidism is a treatable condition.

The Facts about Postmenopausal Bone Loss

Though your bone loss is gradual in the years between achieving peak bone mass and entering menopause, after menopause the loss increases dramatically. The average woman loses up to 3 percent of bone mass a year after menopause. According to the National Osteoporosis Foundation, women can lose up to 20 percent of their bone mass in just the first five to seven years following menopause.

So does that mean that every woman emerges from the first decade of menopause with thin, fragile bones? Certainly not! Remember that the condition of your bones plays a role in preserving their mass, as do a number of other factors, including heredity, environment, diet, and exercise.

All of these facts lead to only one logical conclusion: Every woman—regardless of her age or health—needs to understand her risks for developing osteoporosis and have a sound, ongoing plan for maintaining her bone health. Waiting until you're older or waiting until you've entered menopause to protect yourself against osteoporosis just won't work; by then, you could already be losing the battle against bone loss.

Understanding and Controlling Your Risks

If every woman goes through menopause, why doesn't every woman develop osteoporosis? The risk factors for developing this disease go well beyond age and hormonal production rates. Here are some of the genetic, environmental, and other risk factors for developing this disease:

- **Body makeup:** Women with thin, small frames are at greater risk of suffering excessive bone loss as they age.
- **A family history of osteoporosis:** If other women (or men) in your family developed this disease, your risk for developing it goes up.
- **Caucasian or Asian race:** African-American women have a much lower incidence of postmenopausal osteoporosis than do Northern European and Asian women. However, they still need the same screening for other risk factors.
- **Taking certain medications:** If you've taken steroids (such as prednisone), anticonvulsants, thyroid hormone replacement therapy, or lithium, for more than three months, your risks for developing osteoporosis increase.

- **Eating disorders:** A history of eating disorders such as anorexia or bulimia can increase your risks. Infrequent or irregular periods can be a sign that excessive dieting is resulting in low estrogen levels.
- **Lifestyle choices:** Excess consumption of alcohol, inadequate calcium intake, cigarette smoking, and a lack of exercise all can contribute to the development of osteoporosis over time. If your diet is low in calcium, you're putting yourself at risk for developing the disease.

As you can see, some risk factors are controllable and others aren't. But you have many options available to you for preventing or slowing the progress of osteoporosis. The National Osteoporosis Foundation recommends these four steps for preventing or managing the disease:

- Eat a healthy diet that includes ample supplies of calcium and vitamin D.
- Incorporate weight-bearing exercise, such as walking or weight lifting, in your regular exercise plan (and that means doing these exercises three or more times a week).
- Stop smoking and don't overindulge in alcohol.
- If you're at high risk for osteoporosis, get regular bone density tests.

FACTS

Osteoporosis-related fractures can be killers. In 1991, nearly 300,000 Americans age forty-five and older were hospitalized as a result of hip fractures, and osteoporosis was a contributor to most of these breaks. On average, 24 percent of patients who experience a hip fracture after the age of fifty die within the year that follows their fracture.

Eating for Strong Bones

You already know that your diet plays a big role in your overall health, but a balanced diet rich in calcium and vitamin D is particularly important for preventing or slowing the progress of osteoporosis. Your body stores pounds of calcium in its bones, and calcium is an essential nutrient for all of your body's organs and tissues. Therefore, maintaining

your calcium levels helps keep all of your body—not just its bones—
healthy and fit.

A woman's calcium requirement changes as she ages. Between the
ages of eleven and twenty-four, you should get at least 1,200 milligrams of
calcium every day. You can drop that amount to 800 milligrams per day
from ages twenty-five to fifty. By the time you reach age fifty, you need at
least 1,200 to 1,500 milligrams of calcium every day. (If you're still having
periods or taking estrogen, the lower number will do, but if you're in
menopause and not on estrogen, move up to the higher amount.) What
foods give you the greatest calcium boost? Here are just some examples
(remember to check food product labels):

Food	Milligrams of Calcium
Nonfat, plain yogurt, 1 cup	452
Swiss cheese, 1½ oz.	408
Skim milk, 1 cup	302
Whole milk, 1 cup	291
Sardines, canned with bones, 3 oz.	321
Almonds, ⅓ cup	114
Kale, cooked, 1 cup	179
Spinach, fresh or cooked, ½ cup	122
Macaroni and cheese, 1 cup	362
Tofu, 1 cup	260
Vanilla ice cream, 1 cup	170

But getting plenty of calcium isn't your only dietary weapon against
osteoporosis. Vitamin D doesn't put more calcium into your system, but it
does help your body use the calcium you eat. Your body absorbs vitamin
D from the sun; if you live in a cold or northern climate, or don't spend
much time outdoors, vitamin D added to your calcium supplement will
help your gastrointestinal system absorb the calcium. Women between the
ages of fifty-one and seventy need about 400 units of vitamin D every
day. You can get 25 percent of your daily requirement simply by drinking
an eight-ounce glass of vitamin D-fortified milk every day. Eggs and some

fish, including sardines, mackerel, and herring, contain small amounts of vitamin D.

Don't misunderstand; eating a well-balanced diet with adequate amounts of calcium and vitamin D won't guarantee an osteoporosis-free life. But without question it's the best method available for helping your body prevent or slow the disease.

QUESTIONS?

Can you be a vegetarian and eat a bone-healthy diet?
Yes you can! However, you must eat a well-balanced diet of beans, seeds, grains, and a broad variety of vegetables. Ovo-lacto vegetarians eat eggs and dairy products, and therefore have more access to calcium in their diet. If you eat no dairy products at all, you need to carefully monitor your calcium intake and consider supplements.

Using Calcium and Vitamin Supplements

Although diet is always the best source of vitamins and nutrients, as you approach menopause, you may find that your diet needs some boosters in the form of supplements. Some estimates indicate that most menopausal women eat only about half as much calcium as they require each day. And many women have trouble digesting dairy products, so upping their intake of milk, yogurt, and cheese may not be an option for getting the increased calcium their bones demand.

Calcium supplements are available in a number of forms today, and they can be a great benefit to any woman approaching menopause. Keep these facts in mind when choosing and using calcium supplements:

• The elemental calcium content of any supplement is what matters most. Check the label carefully to make sure the supplement carries the appropriate amount of elemental calcium.
• Choose calcium supplements from reputable makers; check the label to see if the calcium is purified and look for the USP (United States Pharmacopeia) symbol to help guarantee the reliability of the source.

- Calcium works best when you take it in 500 milligram doses, divided over the course of the day.

FACTS

Your body may be intolerant of a fast, sizeable increase of calcium; signs of that intolerance can be indigestion or gas. Try to build slowly toward your full dosage, and if your system continues to have problems, try a different calcium supplement. A calcium-supplemented orange juice may reduce these side effects.

Because vitamin D is available in few nondairy foods, many people need to supplement their daily supply. Most all-purpose vitamins contain a daily dose of vitamin D, as do some calcium supplements. And minerals such as phosphorous and magnesium are important for bone health, too. Again, adequate doses of these are available in most multivitamins.

Remember, a well-balanced diet is always your best source of nutrients, including vitamins and minerals. But as women approach menopause, most find that they need supplements to round out their daily requirements of calcium. As with any health-related plan, however, discuss all dietary and food supplement decisions with your doctor or health care professional before making any changes in your current practices.

Exercising as Prevention

You probably didn't hear it here first, but exercise is an absolute must for a healthy life—and a healthy passage through menopause. Exercise plays a particularly important role in protecting your bones. Studies have shown that weight-bearing exercise builds strong, healthy, resilient bones and can slow the progress of bone loss. Walking, one of the most popular forms of exercise, seems to be particularly helpful in encouraging new bone growth. Exercise not only helps maintain your bones' health but also keeps your joints and muscles flexible and strong. Those improvements alone go a long way toward helping you prevent fractures caused by falls.

Most health care professionals recommend thirty minutes of weight bearing exercise—such as walking or other moderately intense physical activity—three days a week, as part of a total exercise program that also includes aerobic and stretching exercises. If you go with a weight lifting program, make sure you get the help and advice of your health care professional in planning a program that will offer you the maximum benefit and the minimum risk of strain or injury.

Exercise alone won't prevent osteoporosis. But if you combine a sensible exercise program with a well-balanced diet (remember those high levels of calcium and vitamin D) and avoid smoking and excess alcohol consumption, you'll go a long way to preserving your bone health, even after menopause.

Using Estrogen for Bone Health

Diet, exercise, and nutritional supplements can all slow the bone loss your body experiences after menopause, but they can't stop it. However, most doctors agree that estrogen therapy can halt bone loss during this time and may actually contribute to bone growth. Estrogen helps to activate the vitamin D in your body to enhance its ability to absorb calcium. It also promotes the production of collagen in your system that aids in the development of bone strength and flexibility.

Estrogen replacement therapy (ERT) has been shown to reduce bone loss, increase bone density in the spine and hip, and reduce the risk of hip fractures in postmenopausal women. If you are approaching menopause, talk to your health care professional about the benefits and risks of estrogen for the prevention of osteoporosis after menopause. ERT is also beneficial for the heart, eyes, brain, colon, and joints, so try to touch on all these areas with your physician.

FACTS

Calcitonin is the hormone your parathyroid gland produces to help control bone loss. The FDA has approved calcitonin, available in a prescription nasal spray, for treatment—not prevention—of osteoporosis.

Other Options for Slowing Bone Loss

In addition to estrogen, some "designer" estrogens, including raloxifene, and the biphosphonates alendronate and risedronate have been approved by the U.S. Food and Drug Administration (FDA) for the prevention and treatment of postmenopausal osteoporosis. Though these drugs don't share estrogen's other benefits, they may help to maintain bone density, and represent a welcome alternative to estrogen for women who want a sound defense against osteoporosis, but who cannot or choose not to take estrogen in HRT. (See Chapters 11 and 12 for a full discussion of HRT and its alternatives.)

Alendronate, risedronate, and raloxifene have been shown to reduce bone loss, increase bone density, and reduce the risk of fractures, just like estrogen. Raloxifene is among the newest of these designer estrogens, and it may offer some of the most attractive benefits. Raloxifene comes from a relatively new class of drugs called selective estrogen receptor modulators (SERMs) that prevent bone loss. According to the National Osteoporosis Foundation, early tests have shown that raloxifene increases bone mass and, after three years of use, can reduce the risk of spine fractures by about 50 percent.

Whether you choose to use natural estrogens or designer estrogens to prevent postmenopausal bone loss, your doctor or health care professional is your best source of advice and information for making this important decision. But don't depend on either approach as your only solution for staving off bone loss. No matter what type of medications or supplements you take, a healthy diet and regular weight-bearing exercise are important components of your antiosteoporosis arsenal.

CHAPTER 9

Menopause and Sexuality

W omen in perimenopause are often surprised to find their sexual appetites changing. The reasons for shifts in sexual readiness and desire are as complex as human sexuality itself, and include physical, emotional, psychological, and chemical changes natural in a maturing body. By learning more about the potential impact of menopause on your own sexuality, you're better prepared to manage your experience.

A New Sexual Revolution

Popular culture is woven together by an infinite public appetite for sexuality; if you doubt that, just count the number of sexual references you encounter in any evening spent watching television, reading magazines, watching films, or listening to popular radio. Nevertheless, the public fascination with female sexuality has very definite boundaries, and those boundaries are determined by age. So, while the sexual appetites and capabilities of women in their twenties and thirties seem to hold endless fascination for the public at large, that interest flags dramatically when the subject turns to the sex life of women in menopause. And when you do see or hear popular references to the sexuality of the overforty female set, those references are more likely intended to disturb or amuse—not titillate—the viewer or listener.

In the past, many people assumed that women lost their desire for sex as they approached menopause, and that the passage through menopause led inevitably toward the eventual death of the libido. Today, most people know that idea is simply untrue and dismiss it as outdated mythology; still, not everyone understands all of the ways the physical changes of menopause can affect sexuality.

FACTS

A landmark 1986 study by Masters & Johnson (Sex and Aging—Expectations and Reality) found that women can remain sexually active their entire lives with no decline in orgasmic potential, and may become more orgasmic. The study also found that normal changes of sexual response and aging don't equate to decreased sexual functioning.

Thanks to the burgeoning numbers of women moving into midlife today, however, the discussion, research, and medical information on maturing female sexuality has never been richer. Talking about libido with other people is no longer considered taboo. Women can turn to doctors, health care professionals, and books such as this one to educate themselves about exactly what kinds of physical symptoms and changes may affect their sexuality during menopause, and how to maintain optimum sexual health during this time. That understanding paves the way for a sexual revolution as socially significant as the first one these Baby Boomers experienced back in the 1960s—an era of the sexually confident, healthy, and vital midlife woman!

The Physical Facts of Life

If you abandon the idea that sexual problems of midlife are all in the head, the next step toward managing your own maturing sexual health is to understand the facts of life for this stage of your life. So what physical symptoms and changes can interfere with sexual desire and pleasure as menopause approaches? Here are the most common:

- Vaginal dryness
- Pain during penetration
- Reduced response to clitoral stimulation and other sexual stimuli

Some of these changes are absolutely normal parts of the aging process and don't represent alarming signals that sexual life is drawing to a close. Women (and men, for that matter) typically experience a slowdown in their biologic sexual response. Women may take longer to become aroused, for example, and some women report that they have fewer orgasmic contractions and shorter orgasms in general. These changes just mean that lovemaking takes on a new schedule or some new practices—changes that can benefit lovemaking at any age. Other physical changes are transient and treatable, either with medical hormonal therapies or nonhormonal, natural techniques.

But a maturing woman can undergo a number of physical and medical events that can trigger the symptoms and conditions of flagging sexual health, as well. These events include:

- Illnesses, both physical and emotional, including (but not limited to) cardiac problems, hypertension, cancer, bladder disease, depression, and arthritis
- Medications used to treat any of the above illnesses, including some antihypertensives, antidepressants, tranquilizers, and antihistamines
- Medical treatments, such as radiation therapy, chemotherapy, or surgery

Don't get the impression that if you take blood pressure medication or undergo surgery that you're embarking on a life of sexual abstinence. Sexual dysfunction resulting from illness or long-term treatments such as chemotherapy can pass as the illness and treatment side effects fade. A number of alternative medications can replace those that create sexual problems for certain individuals.

Medical causes of female sexual dysfunction are rarely permanent or untreatable. That's why it's important that any woman experiencing any change in her sexual functions talk to her doctor or health care provider. If a medical condition or treatment is contributing to the problem, a health care professional can explain how long the problem may persist, or change treatments or medications that may be triggering it.

Hormones and Sexuality

Let's not forget one of the primary causes for many sexual health issues in perimenopausal and menopausal women—the loss of estrogen that results from the slowdown and eventual cessation of a woman's reproductive cycle. Hormonal imbalances can trigger or exacerbate many of the physical symptoms that can erode a healthy, perimenopausal woman's sex life.

Hormones—especially estrogen—play an important role in your body's sexual response. Estrogen helps to nourish all of your body's tissues, including your vagina, vulva, and urethra. Estrogen also helps keep the clitoris well nourished and responsive; with less estrogen, the clitoris can lose some of its ability to respond to touch.

As your vaginal wall becomes thinner and drier, your vagina can become shorter, narrower, and less elastic. If this vaginal atrophy becomes severe, sex can be quite painful. Lack of lubrication and vaginal walls that just won't give can make sex less appealing—to both the woman, and her partner.

A lack of estrogen will also result in a change in the normal vaginal pH, and lower levels of lactobacillus, the normal bacteria that helps ward off most vaginal infections in reproductive age women. Thus, if your vagina goes through marked changes in pH levels, you may find that you're more susceptible to vaginal infections. These infections can make your vagina feel raw and irritated, create abnormal vaginal discharge, and make sexual intercourse a painful, burning experience. Estrogen replacement therapy can improve vaginal secretions and tone, and can even be used in the form of a vaginal cream for more rapid effects. (Other techniques for maintaining vaginal health are found in "Maintaining Your Sexual Health," later in this chapter.)

Hormones play another critical role in strengthening or diminishing the libido; the sex hormones—estrogen and progesterone—contribute to mood. If you grow anxious, depressed, irritable, or exhausted as a result of hormone deficiencies, your sex life can suffer.

Beyond the Physical Factor

Without question, a woman's psychological and emotional state can trigger many of the physical symptoms associated with aging sexuality. When a woman has low self-esteem or a poor body image, for example, she can have a greatly reduced response to stimulation. Anxiety, sleeplessness, and hot flashes can interfere with a woman's ability to anticipate or enjoy sex and contribute to one or more of the previously listed physical symptoms. Decreased sexual activity itself can lead to diminished sexual desire, pleasure, and response. A woman with a sexually dysfunctional partner—or no partner at all—can be at risk of losing her own sexual health as a result.

FACTS

See "Your Mate May Be Menopausal, Too" in Chapter 1, "Every Woman's Menopause . . . and Yours"; Changes in Libido in Chapter 2, "Understanding the Symptoms of Perimenopause"; and Chapter 17, "Finding Your New Sexuality," which discusses techniques for revitalizing your sex drive.

Any woman knows that her most important responses to sexual stimulation take place in her brain; as a result, any number of conditions or illnesses can impair a woman's libido, including alcoholism, fatigue, depression, and chronic illnesses. It's hard to dispute the fact that our libido is all tangled up in our self-esteem. Perimenopause and natural menopause are transitions associated with aging, and if self-esteem suffers as a result of aging, sexual desire may suffer, too. Our bodies change during perimenopause; that, too, is an undeniable fact. The degree of that change varies, of course, and we have many tools at our disposal to help maintain our physical health and vitality as we grow older. But women who combat weight gain, fatigue, depression, and feelings of isolation during perimenopause are at risk for suffering from flagging sexual desire, as well.

And our partners—male or female—are changing, too. Two women going through perimenopause at the same time may experience a multitude of sexual issues as they try to maintain their sexual closeness as each rides her own roller coaster of menopausal symptoms. Men can experience a loss of sexual potency and desire as they age, and that can have a direct impact on the sexual confidence and health of their partners. If a sexual partner seems uninterested in sex or unable to sustain an erection or become aroused, it's easy for the other partner to feel inadequate, undesirable, and definitely unsexy. It's also not easy to feel good about yourself if your husband or partner decides to dump you for a trophy wife or neglects you to chase after a mistress.

You have an important opportunity to improve your sex life during perimenopause. This time of transition encourages women to reassess their lives, their relationships, and their attitudes toward living. You have a wide variety of physical and psychological tools available to you to help take your sexuality to new heights as your body enjoys sex for reasons that have nothing to do with reproduction.

Maintaining Your Sexual Health

Now, you might read the preceding paragraphs and think, "I'm doomed to lose my sexuality, because I (along with every other woman living on this planet) have one of these conditions, use some of these medications, or am experiencing some of these issues." But you can toss those fears away, right now. Most of the events, issues, treatments, and so on listed above can—but may not necessarily—lead to temporary sexual dysfunction. Nearly every symptom or problem that affects your sexual health is treatable, reversible, or even avoidable. But, as with any area of your health maintenance, you can't count on someone else—your doctor, minister, therapist, or partner—to protect and manage your sexual health. That job is yours.

FACTS

In a survey of forty-five- to sixty-five-year-old men and women conducted in 2001 by *Newsweek* magazine, 30 percent of women and 34 percent of men surveyed thought sex is more enjoyable for people their age than for younger people, 40 percent of women and 47 percent of men said it was "about the same," while only 16 percent and 12 percent (respectively) thought sex "less enjoyable" with age.

If you, like the vast majority of men and women in this country, intend to remain sexually active throughout a long and healthy life, what can you do to ensure that you maintain your sexual health through the years ahead? Later chapters talk about specific ideas for exploring and enhancing your new sexuality and for treating causes of sexual dysfunction. Chapters 11 and 12, for example, discuss hormone replacement therapy and its alternatives—common and very effective methods for treating a wide range of physical (and emotional) symptoms that impair sexual response and functions. And Chapter 17 covers the ways you can keep your sex drive alive and happy during and well after menopause. But before you begin any of those treatment or practice alternatives, you have four very basic tools at your disposal for monitoring and maintaining your sexual health:

- Monitor your sexual health and pay attention to changes in your sexual responses and feelings
- Maintain an open dialog with your health care professional about sexual problems and solutions
- Maintain your vaginal health
- Use appropriate birth control methods while still in perimenopause

Listen to Your Sexual Self

One of the most important things you can do to maintain your sexual health is to pay attention to what your body and mind are telling you about your feelings about your sexuality, your attitude toward sex in general, and your evolving sexual response. Your sexuality evolves with the rest of you, and the entire package has changed dramatically over past twenty years. To illustrate, just choose an answer to this question:

My idea of a great evening is:
a. Dancing and drinking 'til dawn in a local nightspot
b. Getting "hit on" and picked up in a bar
c. Going out on a first date
d. Sitting at home reading, watching television, or doing anything else that enables me to wear sweatpants without sweating

Many of those who choose D (and that's many of us over the age of forty), wouldn't have chosen it twenty years ago. And that's not a sign of age—it's a sign of maturity. Your sexual interests and responses change, too; sexual techniques you used to enjoy might have lost some—or all—of their appeal over time. As your sexual tastes evolve, you can find totally new and different ways to enjoy sex, and that's just one of the benefits of seniority.

Don't try to force yourself into a sexuality that doesn't fit; some people have strong libidos and sex drives; others don't. Think about your sexuality and accept the sexual person you are, but don't try to settle for less or berate yourself because you don't want more. Be honest with your sexual self.

But if you suddenly realize that sex no longer holds any interest for you; or that you don't like your body enough to share it in sexual relations with anyone; or that it's just too painful, awkward, difficult, or otherwise unpleasant to "mess with" sex, you need to stop and ask yourself when—and why—these feelings arose in you. You're too young (at any age) to just walk away from a sexually fulfilling life.

If you find your interest in sex or your ability to respond to sexual stimulation fading dramatically, you shouldn't chalk it up to maturity. Enjoying your sexuality is part of leading a healthy, well-rounded life. And a sudden or severe loss of interest in sex can signal other problems—both emotional and physical—that can grow worse as time goes by. Remember, the old saying "use it or lose it" is frequently applied to sexuality. Long periods of abstinence can undermine your ability to become aroused, and lack of sexual activity can promote vaginal atrophy and a diminished response to sexual stimulation.

In any event, you aren't better off just forgetting about it. You deserve and benefit from a healthy, active sexual self—whether you have a partner or not. Even single, older women should be able to feel sexually aroused by certain images—whether it's a good-looking actor, an advertisement for lingerie, or a steamy passage in a book. If you aren't enjoying (or even thinking about) sex, you have many options for regaining your sexual enjoyment—whether that involves exploring new sexual techniques, examining your attitudes about your sexuality, or investigating possible medical causes for your diminishing sexual interests or abilities.

Let's Talk about S-E-X

As your sexuality matures with you, you might experience any or all of the problems or issues discussed in this chapter. And, in most cases, you may need to talk to a medical professional, therapist, or other counselor or consultant to find the best resolution for those problems. If you aren't comfortable discussing medical or emotional aspects of your sexuality or sexual health, that discomfort can make your situation seem even more frustrating and hopeless. Your ability to talk about issues—ranging from painful intercourse to a lack of response to stimulation—is crucial to establish a trusting relationship with your health care provider, and to become comfortable discussing your sexual health with that person.

Talking to a professional can help. If a lack of interest in sex is a side effect of a growing sense of depression and isolation, a counselor, friend, or therapist may be able to help you explore and resolve the source of those feelings. If sex is physically less enjoyable—even painful--your gynecologist, internist, or other health care provider can prescribe medications, exercises, or other treatments to resolve the source of those problems.

SSENTIALS As the population ages, health care professionals are spending more time dealing with issues of mature sexuality. Doctors, nurses, and therapists are aware that many patients have difficulty discussing sexual problems and might need sensitive guidance in these discussions, and therefore, closely follow developments in both treatments for sexual problems.

So, the first step in resolving issues of sexual health is to notice when they arise. The second step is to talk to the appropriate professional to get the right kind of medical, psychological, or other therapeutic treatment to help resolve the issues. Begin by talking to the health care professional or counselor you trust most. If that person can't provide the professional assistance you need, he or she can refer you to the appropriate source for that help.

Stay Healthy

Chapter 17, "Finding Your New Sexuality," offers some specific ideas for exploring new sexual techniques, re-evaluating your sexual interests, and maintaining a healthy, open attitude toward your sexuality. But a primary physical component of an active, healthy sexuality is a healthy vagina. Your vagina is maturing along with the rest of your body, and it's worth your while to pay some special attention to caring for this sensitive (and vital) part of your body. Don't worry—you don't need a special course in maintenance and repair to keep this part of your sexual being in order. Some very simple techniques and common-sense practices can help you maintain your vaginal health as you journey through menopause.

First, if your sexual life involves new partners, always practice safe sex. This isn't the 1960s, and casual, unprotected sex with strangers never again will be in fashion. Don't count on your judgment or gut reaction to determine whether or not someone's infected with AIDS or other sexually transmitted diseases (STDs). Assume that they are—no matter who they are—and don't allow a sexual partner's semen, blood, or other body fluids to come in contact with your vagina, anus, or mouth. Your vaginal tissues are becoming thinner and easier to tear, and your immune system might be stressed by shifting hormone levels. That puts you more at risk than ever for contracting a sexually transmitted disease. Talk to your partner about his or her sexual history, use condoms, and get blood tests. Safe sex practices may not seem sexy, but they're basic to survival.

Next, take steps to reduce vaginal dryness. Your vaginal secretions diminish along with your estrogen level, which can contribute to dry, inflexible vaginal tissues and painful intercourse. Your vagina's pH balance will shift with your hormone levels, too, and that can contribute to increased irritation and bacterial infections. Estrogen replacement is one way to combat vaginal dryness, but it's not the only method for keeping vaginal tissues moist and pliant.

FACTS

Sexual activity (with or without a partner) is one of the most pleasant methods for encouraging healthy, moist vaginal tissues. When you become sexually aroused, more blood flows to your vaginal tissues, stimulating the release of your vagina's natural lubricants. Frequent arousal is good for you.

Over-the-counter vaginal moisturizers such as Astroglide, K-Y Jelly, and Vagisil Moisturizer can help fight off dryness. (Ask your doctor or pharmacist for other vaginal moisturizing products.) Avoid vaginal deodorizers and deodorized products, scented toilet tissues, and chemical-laden bath soaps and soaks. Perfumes and chemicals can further upset the pH balance in your vagina and contribute to local irritation and dryness. Be sure to drink plenty of water and eat a diet rich in fruit, whole grains, and vegetables (a good idea for any time of life). Water hydrates all of your cells; drink between thirty-two and sixty-four ounces every day to keep you skin, hair, bones, and other body tissues fully moisturized.

Don't Forget about Birth Control

Remember, until you have gone for twelve months without a period or until your doctor or health care provider has run appropriate blood tests to determine the levels of hormones your body is producing, you could ovulate and, therefore, become pregnant after sexual activity. Many women stop using birth control after they've missed four or five periods and feel that they're no longer fertile. That's a mistake; a surprise pregnancy in your midforties can be a tremendous problem for both you and your partner. Again, be smart, and use contraceptives for a year after your last period.

CHAPTER 10

Your Mind, Mood, and Emotional Health

Your emotional health and physical health are closely linked. This connection between them is never more keenly felt than during menopause and the years immediately preceding and following it. Many women experience a series of physical, chemical, and social changes during perimenopause that can shake their self-confidence and threaten their emotional health. But you have a remarkable ability to control the speed and severity of those changes.

Where Did It Go?

If you're nearing age fifty and you haven't yet begun to experience periodic memory lapses, consider yourself lucky. The busier and more stressful life becomes, the easier it is to misplace car keys, forget an associate's name, lose track of the point you were about to make, and remember the title of that movie starring, "That guy with the eyebrows—you know the one who married that woman who was in the soap opera for so many years . . . the one who's dead now . . . shoot, it's on the tip of my tongue." Sound familiar? As one fifty-something friend once said, "It takes three middle-aged people to tell any one story." Multiple events challenge the memory at middle age; some of these challenges stem from the inevitable physical changes of age, and many of them are not yet fully understood by the scientific and medical communities. Though many women wonder if they're showing the first signs of Alzheimer's, the vast majority of memory loss problems are natural—and sometimes transient—responses to the effects of age, menopausal hormone changes, stress, and a busy, changing life.

FACTS

Alzheimer's disease is more common in women than in men, and it strikes women at an earlier age. The symptoms, which include memory loss, diminished language and motor skills, and an inability to recognize people or objects, appear gradually and worsen with age. The causes of Alzheimer's are still under investigation.

Many women report an increase in forgetfulness, memory loss, and mental clarity during perimenopause. Because hormones tend to fluctuate dramatically during perimenopause, estrogen deficiency used to be the culprit most often blamed for changes in memory functions. But recent studies, such as the Seattle Midlife Women's Health Study, conducted by the University of Washington in 2000, dispute that notion. In that study, researchers found that neither the age nor the perimenopausal stage of the women studied were linked to any diminishment of the women's mental functions. In fact, the study found that younger women and women undergoing hormone therapy were more likely than midlife women to report problems with memory loss.

Many types of memory loss at midlife are attributable to other, more combatable factors, such as overwork, stress, anxiety, and depression. The Seattle study found that physical health, emotional factors, and stress accounted for almost half of the memory loss noted in participants. Depression and high levels of stress played a key role in short-term memory degradation. Among participants in the study, only 24 percent of memory loss was attributed to the physical effects of aging.

ESSENTIALS

Although you don't have to fear that your brain will shrink up like a walnut when you hit fifty, real physical changes in it can begin at this time, and you may begin to feel their impact on your short-term memory, attention span, and other thinking processes. Chapter 19, "Keeping Your Mind Sharp," offers some simple techniques for keeping your mental edge as you move toward and through menopause.

Most medical and scientific authorities agree that age results in subtle changes in anyone's ability to think clearly and quickly, but that doesn't link memory loss to menopause; causes for these mental lapses are tied more closely to the brain than the ovaries. First, the human brain shrinks after age fifty, due to a loss of water content. That shrinkage doesn't necessarily impair memory, of course, but a loss of volume in the frontal lobes can. Some neuroscientists say that the frontal lobes can shrink as much as 30 percent between the ages of fifty and ninety. Because the frontal lobes are so important to complex thinking, losses in that area of the brain can impair your ability to reason things out, maintain attention span, multitask, and use your best judgment.

And the brain's hippocampus can lose some of its capabilities with age, too. This part of the brain is responsible for creating, storing, and retrieving memory, and scientists now think it can lose a portion of those abilities with age. A slowing of mental processes accounts for many of the cognitive changes that you perceive with age. In other words, the information is all there and your brain can retrieve it—that retrieval process just takes longer than it used to. Metabolic changes and a diminished number of brain signal transmitter neurons (dendrites) contribute to the slowdown.

Menopause and Depression

Are you certain to suffer from depression as you approach menopause? No, no, no—and absolutely not! Many women report that midlife brings them a confidence, serenity, and inner peace that they've never before experienced. In fact, although women are more prone to depression than men (at rates two to three times higher), women in their childbearing years—years often spent simultaneously raising children and establishing careers—are much more likely to develop depression than are women in menopause.

Nevertheless, nearly 25 percent of all women will suffer from a type of depression at some time during their lives. And women who have a family or personal history of depression are more at-risk for suffering from depression during perimenopause. The connection between this period of transition and depression can be both physical and emotional. But to better understand that connection, you first need to understand exactly what depression is—and how it differs from mood swings and minor bouts of "the blues."

FACTS

Mood swings are characterized by strong and sometimes rapidly changing emotional events. Women approaching menopause often (but not always) report anxiety and panic attacks, bouts of sadness, or unexplained surges of elation. These emotional swings tend to be erratic and transient, not long-lived facts of life for perimenopausal women. (Mood swings and perimenopause are covered in Chapter 2.)

What Is Depression?

The term depression is one you hear frequently. It's not unusual for people to say they're depressed by the weather, their jobs, their haircuts, their prospects for dinner, or the night's television lineup. But there's a world of difference between these passing feelings of disappointment, dissatisfaction, or sadness, and an ongoing state of major depression. For all of the overwrought "depressions" you hear about every day, true depression is a real problem faced by hundreds of thousands of people in our society. According to the *Journal of the American Medical Association*, between 5 and 10 percent of the U.S. population experiences major depression; and nearly 25 percent of all women will suffer from depression at some point during their lives.

Many women in perimenopause have minor mood problems that may include insomnia, anxiety, and irritability. But when these problems become severe or long-standing, these women can develop major depression. Major depression is an illness that prevents sufferers from working, eating, sleeping, studying, and enjoying a full, normal life and range of moods. Major depression typically results from changes in brain chemistry; therefore, even though it can occur once in a lifetime, many people who suffer from major depression experience it several times.

Another, less severe, type of depression is known as dysthymia. The symptoms of dysthymia are similar to those of major depression and may be chronic and long-term, but they aren't disabling. Finally, bipolar disorder (manic-depressive illness) is another kind of depression. People suffering from a bipolar disorder experience extreme mood shifts that swing wildly between manic highs and depressed lows.

ESSENTIALS

If you suffer from low self-esteem, feel overwhelmed by stress, or have a persistently pessimistic attitude toward life, you might be at risk for developing depression. Scientists continue to study the causes of depression, to determine whether these types of feelings are an indicator that you're prone to depression, or whether these feelings can actually trigger the illness.

Depression makes itself known to each individual in unique ways, but some symptoms are typical of the disease. The National Institute of Mental Health provides a list of common symptoms of depression (though it notes that few people suffer all of them). Here are some of those symptoms:

- Feeling persistently sad, anxious, empty, hopeless, or pessimistic
- A strong sense of impending doom, with no idea what form this awful event might take or why it will happen

- A loss of interest in hobbies or activities you once enjoyed (including sex)
- Feeling guilty, worthless, or helpless
- Losing energy and feeling fatigued and slowed down
- Suffering from insomnia, early morning awakening, or oversleeping
- Experiencing a dramatic change in appetite or weight
- Difficulty concentrating, remembering, or making decisions
- Thoughts of suicide and death or suicide attempts
- Feeling restless and irritable
- Suffering from persistent physical symptoms (headache, pain, digestive disorders) that don't respond to treatment.

FACTS

Many types of medical, psychotherapeutic, and alternative treatment options can help you avoid and overcome depression. To find out about those options and how to play a role in your own battle with depression, anxiety, and moodiness, see Chapter 18.

The Causes of Depression

No one cause is at the source of every case of depression, but it usually is associated with a change in the brain's structure or functions. Sometimes a vulnerability to depression is genetically inherited, but depression can be brought on by physical changes resulting from stress, injury, an accident, or a severe emotional event. If an individual feels at the mercy of a disease or illness, he or she can fall into depression. Severe illnesses such as heart attack, stroke, and cancer can lead to depression, as can progressive illnesses such as Parkinson's disease. Financial problems, the death of a loved one, the loss of a job, a parent's illness, the departure of grown children, and other stressful changes to a daily routine also can push people into depression. Even a change of address or an abrupt change in a close circle of friends can trigger the onset of a depression that's been building over time. Finally, hormonal shifts, such as those women experience in pregnancy, perimenopause, and menopause, can also contribute to depression in women.

If you consider all of these potential triggers, you easily can see how some women might suffer from depression during perimenopause. Menopause itself doesn't cause these cases of depression, but the hormonal changes of perimenopause can join with other natural life events of middle age to contribute to a depressed state. Women who have suffered in the past from depression or who have experienced severe PMS seem to be especially vulnerable to depression during perimenopause.

As you approach menopause, consider your risks for depression. Do you have a family history of depression? Have you suffered from severe PMS or postpartum depression earlier in your life? If you have a predisposition to this illness, don't ignore feelings of depression that arise as you near the age of menopause. Talk to your doctor, therapist, or other health care professional about your concerns early; don't let depression build; it's much easier to treat earlier than later.

Insomnia and Its Role in Menopause

Insomnia is a typical symptom of perimenopause, and it plays an active cause-and-effect role in several other perimenopausal conditions. Night sweats and panic attacks, for example, can contribute to insomnia. Long-term insomnia can contribute to heightened anxiety and feelings of fatigue, moodiness, and irritability. When women don't get enough rest, they can have difficulty with concentration, focus, and memory, and their overall physical and mental health can suffer.

Insomnia—a condition characterized by an inadequate amount or poor quality of sleep occurring three or more nights a week—isn't just a concern of menopausal women, of course; as a nation, the United States has entered a time of greater sleeplessness than perhaps ever before. The National Sleep Foundation (an independent, nonprofit organization) released the results of its own national sleep survey in 2001; that survey revealed that 60 percent of American adults report some sort of sleep problem, and most say they were able to get more sleep in the past (as little as five years earlier) than at the time of the survey.

With nearly 40 million people in the United States suffering from some sort of sleep disorder, it's a given that a large number of perimenopausal and menopausal women are among them. In fact, the National Sleep Foundation's 1998 poll, Women and Sleep, found that the average woman between the ages of thirty and sixty sleeps only six hours and forty-one minutes a night during the workweek. "Women are probably the most sleep-deprived creatures on earth," according to Joyce A. Walsleben, Ph.D., director of the Sleep Disorders Center at the New York University School of Medicine. Good, restful sleep is essential to physical and mental well-being, so every woman approaching menopause should understand the connection between her life phase and her sleep cycles, so she can be prepared to overcome sleep problems that might develop during this time.

FACTS

Six in ten adults in the United States say they experience frequent sleep problems. In the National Sleep Survey of 2001, a high percentage of those with certain health problems common to perimenopause experienced sleep problems, including depression (83 percent), nighttime heartburn (82 percent), and hypertension (79 percent).

Hormonal Imbalances and Sleeplessness

Remember when you were a teenager and could—if allowed—sleep past noon? For most women approaching menopause, that capacity for endless sleep is only a distant memory. A woman's hormonal balance affects her ability to sleep throughout her adult life; many women experience sleep disturbances during menstruation, pregnancy, and in perimenopause and menopause.

Women who experience PMS (premenstrual syndrome) often report sleeping difficulties during that same, late phase of the menstrual cycle (Days 22 through 28). The physical symptoms of PMS include bloating, headache, moodiness, and cramping—all of which can contribute to sleeplessness. But women with PMS report a range of sleep problems in addition to insomnia, including hypersomnia (a condition in which you sleep too much) and daytime sleepiness. As women who have a history of PMS approach menopause, those symptoms can become even more severe.

FACTS

Women who are healthy sleepers spend 15 to 20 percent of their sleeping hours in deep sleep. Some research has suggested that women who have PMS may spend only 5 percent of their sleeping hours in deep sleep all month long.

Women in menopause report more sleep disorders than women in any other age group. Many sleep problems in perimenopause are caused by other symptoms of diminishing hormones, including hot flashes and night sweats. Though these problems may not diminish the length of a woman's sleep cycle, they can disrupt sleep frequently enough to cause fatigue and sleepiness throughout the following day. In the NSF poll, women reported that hot flashes contributed to their sleep disturbances at least five days a month.

Many doctors recommend hormone replacement therapy (HRT) or alternative treatments to combat many of the symptoms of perimenopause and menopause, including sleeplessness. (See Chapters 11 and 12.)

The Source of Sleep Problems

Hormonal imbalances aren't the only cause of sleep disruption for women in perimenopause and menopause. Depression and anxiety are common contributors to sleeplessness, and these problems are factors for some perimenopausal women. Remember, these problems feed each other. The less rested you are, the more powerful your negative feelings become, and the less able you are to see your way through them. Stress—an enemy of women at any age—can also severely inhibit your ability to enjoy deep, restful sleep. A late-night trip to the bathroom, for example, may be followed by hours of sleeplessness brought on by stress-induced worry. If you awaken due to pain, or have a tendency to "snap" awake at four A.M. for no good reason, and lie in bed worrying about vague concerns or relatively inconsequential issues until the alarm goes off at seven A.M., stress is playing a role in your sleep disturbance. All of these triggers can combine to create a powerful enemy of your good health as you approach and pass through menopause.

FACTS

Rapid Eye Movement (REM) sleep is the most active sleep state—the one in which dreams occur. Scientists divide non-REM sleep (about 80 percent of total sleep) into four stages. In each stage, brain waves grow larger and slower. After the fourth stage, the deepest period of sleep, the brain waves reverse the pattern; sleep progresses toward its lightest stage, REM sleep. Typically, the cycle takes about ninety minutes.

Chapter 18 offers you some valuable techniques for recognizing and combating problems that can contribute to (and feed off) sleeplessness. But acknowledging that sleep disturbance is part of this overall pattern is an important first step in any treatment. The next critical step is to talk with a doctor, counselor, or other health professional about these problems and their solution.

Your sleep problems may have nothing to do with stress, anxiety, or tension, but could have physical sources. One in four women over fifty, for example, suffers from sleep apnea, a sleep disorder in which the sleeper stops breathing for frequent, short periods throughout the night. Snoring and daytime sleepiness are clues that you might be suffering from sleep apnea. Snoring isn't just something men do. It can increase with weight gain—particularly when you gain weight around your neck. If you have a problem with daytime sleepiness and your partner complains that your snoring is becoming louder and more pronounced, see your doctor. Sleep apnea is associated with other medical problems, including high blood pressure and cardiovascular disease, so it isn't something to blow off (so to speak).

More women than men suffer pain-related sleep problems. Pain from arthritis, migraine headaches, tension, chronic fatigue syndrome, and fibromyalgia have been linked to sleep disruption in women. Pain can make falling asleep and sleeping through the night more difficult, but many people fail to report (or recognize) sleeplessness as a problem. If pain is interrupting your sleep, ask your health care professional about your pain management options.

If your partner is a heavy snorer or has other risk factors for sleep apnea, his or her symptoms could cause sleep problems for both of you. Your primary care physician can refer you to a sleep-study medical center that can help diagnose the problem and recommend treatment.

Travel can wreak havoc with sleep quality and quantity, too. Many menopausal and perimenopausal women are in professional positions that require them to travel frequently. Hopping from time zone to time zone, spending long hours in airports and on planes, and sleeping in one hotel after another can seriously damage the quality and quantity of anyone's sleep. If you're already dealing with fluctuating hormones and subsequent hot flashes, night sweats, and periodic anxiety attacks, this kind of disruption can make your sleep problems even more severe.

Is Your Lifestyle Keeping You Awake?

Simple lifestyle choices may be at the root of many sleep disturbances. Although you may be following the same practices you've followed for years, as your body changes in perimenopause and menopause, you may have to become more protective of your body's natural ability to sleep. Here are some of the most common daily habits that can interfere with good, restful sleep:

- **Alcohol:** You may think a nightcap will help you sleep, but it probably won't. Drinking alcohol right before bedtime may help you fall asleep, but it's also likely to wake you up hours before you're ready to rise. Avoid alcohol for at least two to four hours before heading for bed.

- **Caffeine:** Caffeine in coffee, tea, chocolate, or sodas can stimulate your brain and make it difficult for you to go to sleep and stay asleep. Limit the amount of caffeine you consume during the day, and confine that consumption to the morning or early afternoon hours. Or cut out the caffeine altogether by switching to decaf drinks or mineral water.

- **Exercising at night:** Yes, exercise is essential for good health and it's a powerful mind and body stimulant. Exercise regularly to help put your body on a natural schedule, but don't exercise in the two to three hours before bedtime.

- **Smoking:** Nicotine is a stimulant. As you've read in nearly every chapter of this book, your good health requires that you quit altogether. If you continue to smoke, however, stop at least two to three hours before bedtime.

- **Your sleep environment:** If your partner snores; if your cat or dog walks all over you through the night; if your room is too hot, too cold, too noisy, or too bright, you won't sleep well and that means you'll be less healthy. Keep the sleeping room temperature between 65 and 70 degrees. Use light-blocking window shades or wear a sleep mask. Close the doors and windows to block out sound; play calm, soothing music with the device set to shut off automatically. And finally, consider sleeping apart from disruptive sleep partners of any species (a difficult step, but perhaps essential).

FACTS

Now may be the right time to get your sleep on schedule. Your body likes schedules, and if you can train it to go to sleep and wake up at the same time every day, you may enjoy deeper, more restful sleep. And don't linger in bed when you've had enough sleep. Try to rise at the same time every day—even on weekends.

Putting Sleep Disorders to Rest

You can't control your body's evolution, and you probably aren't willing to tell your boss, "No travel until after menopause," so what can you do?

The most important way to promote and protect healthy sleep patterns is to pay attention to sleep problems when they arise and then take action to resolve them. If the lifestyle changes suggested in the preceding section don't alleviate your sleep problems, seek professional help to resolve them. Although polls report that many people describe sleep problems as common experiences, many of those same people will say that they don't suffer from sleep disorders. You may think that missing an hour or two of sleep now and then isn't a problem, but you're probably wrong. If you aren't getting enough sleep—and that means at least eight hours a day for most adults—your physical and emotional health will suffer.

So, if you have trouble falling asleep or are awakening frequently during the night, and none of the lifestyle changes you've made have helped, talk to a health care professional. You have a number of options for resolving sleep problems, including changing your diet, exercise schedule, medications, hormone replacement therapy, relaxation techniques, biofeedback, and psychological counseling. Though sleep disturbances may be a short episode in your passage to menopause, you shouldn't allow them to get the upper hand—for any length of time. Insomnia, anxiety, and fatigue go hand in hand, but they don't have to grab hold of you during perimenopause and menopause. Protect your sleep, so you can protect your health.

CHAPTER 11

Understanding Hormones and HRT

Hormone Replacement Therapy (HRT) has been in place for over fifty years, and though it continues to be the focus of much research and scientific debate, it remains the most studied, respected, and commonly used form of treatment for menopausal symptoms and long-term health implications of menopause. However, HRT does have risks, and it may not be right for everyone.

The Role of Hormones in Your Health

Nearly every preceding chapter of this book offers some information about hormones—their role in your body and the impact of fluctuating hormone levels on your health. But as you prepare to move into the discussion of HRT, it's important that you remember a few of the more important facts about hormones. For example, though your body produces a number of hormones, three hormones play leading roles in your reproductive cycle—estrogen, progesterone, and androgens. All three of these hormones can be used in HRT, and therefore continue to play a role in your health from puberty through your mature years.

FACTS

A 1997 study of women physicians in the United States showed that nearly 48 percent of the physicians studied used HRT. This study, reported in the *Annals of Internal Medicine*, revealed that doctors aren't just recommending HRT—many are using it themselves.

Because hormones are such an important and widely used tool for controlling menopausal symptoms, including hot flashes, night sweats, mood swings, vaginal atrophy, and later, bone loss and deteriorating vision, they are the subject of constant, ongoing medical research. As a result, rarely a month passes that we don't hear of some new development in their use, or some new question regarding their safety or efficacy. As this book goes to press, you can assume that new developments will be emerging, and new information will continue to come to light long after you read these words. In order for you to make decisions based on the best information at hand, however, you need a fundamental understanding of these basic sex hormones and how and why they're used in HRT. The sections that follow give you this basic information. Use it as a platform for a continued discussion with your doctor or other health care provider. If your physician doesn't seem receptive to this type of interaction, now is the time to seek a second opinion.

Estrogen and Its Use in HRT

Estrogen is a growth hormone that stimulates the development of adult sex organs during puberty. At puberty, estrogen promotes development of a woman's breasts and hips with what we think of as natural fat deposits and the resulting contours. Estrogen helps retain calcium in bones, a function that keeps bones strong and whole during childbearing years. It also regulates the balance of HDL and LDL cholesterol in the bloodstream and helps lower your body's total cholesterol level. (See Heart Disease and Menopause in Chapter 6.) Estrogen aids other body functions, such as regulating blood sugar levels and emotional balance. Here are some other important benefits of estrogen:

- Estrogen helps keep skin supple and elastic through its nonstop job of replacing dead cells and maintaining proper collagen structure (the basic structural component of skin and supporting structures).
- Estrogen promotes healthy, well-nourished vaginal tissue to help maintain flexible, moist, and elastic vaginal walls.
- Estrogen may help strengthen the brain's blood supply and therefore aid in the protection of memory and cognitive functions.
- Estrogen helps keep all of your body's cells and muscles healthy and well-toned.

Your body doesn't stop producing estrogen when you stop ovulating, but it produces dramatically lower levels of estrogen as your ovarian function declines. The amount of hormones your ovaries are able to secrete gradually diminishes in your late forties, so your body produces lower amounts of estrogen and other hormones. In the early stages of perimenopause, the pituitary gland in the brain produces its own hormones to try to stimulate the ovaries to produce more estrogen, and it works, for a while. The ovaries occasionally are able to give up enough estrogen to trigger a menstrual period. However, in this transition phase a woman may experience widely fluctuating levels of estrogen for a number of years, until the ovaries shut down completely. The body continues to produce small amounts of estrogen, but only at about 25 percent or less of its premenopause rate—levels too small to support the hormone's age-defying functions in the body.

Estrogen is used in HRT to:

- Diminish hot flashes
- Keep the vaginal walls supple, moist, and well nourished
- Maintain or even increase bone density
- Improve blood cholesterol levels, stimulate blood circulation, and keep the arteries healthy, dilated, and plaque-free to help protect against heart disease
- Help alleviate urinary tract problems and diminish stress and urge incontinence
- Help protect cognitive function
- Lower the risk of age-related macular degeneration of the eye and glaucoma
- Lower the risk of rheumatoid arthritis and Parkinson's disease

FACTS

Estrogen use may aid memory and decrease susceptibility to Alzheimer's disease, though more study is needed to determine this effect. Most studies show that estrogen users who develop Alzheimer's have a delayed onset, compared to the general population, and a lowered severity of the disease.

Estrogen's powerful benefits have resulted in its use in HRT for more than fifty years. In the 1950s and 1960s, many doctors prescribed unopposed estrogen replacement, meaning that the woman received estrogen alone, without the balancing effects of the hormone progesterone, even if she had an intact uterus. But later studies revealed that estrogen given alone could result in the development of endometrial cancer (cancer of the uterine lining), so HRT today almost always involves some combination of estrogen, progesterone, and in some cases, androgens such as testosterone. If a woman has had a hysterectomy, she doesn't need to worry about endometrial cancer, so her HRT prescription should involve only estrogen—a treatment known as ERT, or Estrogen Replacement Therapy.

Estrogens offer many health benefits, but these powerful hormones can have some negative effects. Estrogen can contribute to the ocurrence of blood clots in the deep veins of the legs or the lungs of women who have a history of these problems. If you are considering HRT, and you don't know your family's medical history, now is the time to ask about it. If any of your immediate relatives suffers (or suffered) from blood clots not caused by a predisposing risk factor such as pregnancy, prolonged bed rest, recovery from a motor vehicle accident, and so on, you need to report that information to your doctor or health care professional. A family history of such blood clots could indicate that you, too, carry a risk for the condition; your health care worker will use that information to determine whether he or she can recommend HRT for treatment of your perimenopausal symptoms.

If you have your uterus, your health care professional won't prescribe unopposed estrogen for treatment of menopausal symptoms. Be aware, however, that if you self-medicate with plant estrogens (phytoestrogens) from soy foods or supplements, you may be giving your body unopposed estrogens. Talk to your health care provider about any and all supplements and vitamins you take on a regular basis.

As you progress through perimenopause, your body's hormonal changes take place over a period of months or years, giving your system time to adjust to gradually declining hormone levels. If you go through an induced menopause, such as follows the surgical removal of the ovaries, your menopause will be immediate and, very likely, dramatic in its physical impact. In those cases, your doctor or health care provider is likely to recommend some form of estrogen replacement to help your body through the transition.

Progesterone and Its Use in HRT

Progesterone is an important hormone, though its benefits and impact may seem less dramatic than those of estrogen. Normally, your ovaries produce progesterone in the process of ovulation, so most women in their reproductive years that report having regular menstrual cycles would be expected to have normal progesterone levels. Progesterone has a counterbalancing, stabilizing impact on tissue growth; progesterone helps keep the growth of your uterine lining (endometrium) in check, for example, thereby limiting the quantity of your menstrual blood flow. In your childbearing years, progesterone also promotes the development of nutrients in the uterus, breasts, and fallopian tubes to prepare your body for growing an embryo and bearing a child.

FACTS

Some studies have shown that women who take estrogen and progestin in a combined HRT program have a lower incidence of endometrial cancer than do women who take no hormones at all.

Your progesterone levels drop dramatically when you stop ovulating. Because a woman's body produces the majority of its progesterone during the second half of the ovulatory cycle, if you don't ovulate, your progesterone supply falls. Because progesterone's most important effect in your body is its estrogen-balancing capabilities, most HRT prescriptions for women who still have a uterus include some type of progestin, a pharmaceutically prepared form of the naturally occurring hormone progesterone.

Progestin serves several important purposes in HRT. It helps to mediate the growth-stimulating functions of estrogen, so it reduces the risk of endometrial cancer for women who still have their uterus. In spite of its critical importance for balancing the effects of estrogen in HRT, however, progestin has its drawbacks. Some women experience breast tenderness and water retention when taking progestin with estrogen in an HRT regimen. Other women find that some forms of progestin aggravate mood swings. And many forms of progestin can diminish the heart-healthy effects of estrogen, which is why doctors don't include progestin therapy in HRT if a woman has had a hysterectomy.

For these reasons, doctors and health care providers monitor HRT patients carefully to determine which progestin type and delivery technique works best for each individual. If you have a medical history of high cholesterol or high cholesterol fractions, such as LDL (the "bad" cholesterol) or triglycerides, discuss this history with your doctor before deciding on an HRT prescription.

FACTS

More than half of the women who experience irregular spotting or bleeding after beginning an HRT regimen that includes progestin stop bleeding completely after six months; 80 percent stop bleeding within a year. Continued bleeding (after one year) may indicate a problem with the lining of the uterus, rather than a reaction to HRT. (See "Fibroids, Polyps, and Other Sources of Heavy or Irregular Bleeding" in Chapter 6.)

A number of different types of progestins are available, including:

- Medroxyprogesterone acetate (MPA), used in brand names such as Provera, Cycrin, Amen, and found in estrogen combination compounds such as PremPro and PremPhase
- Norethindrone or other 19-nortestosterone derivatives in estrogen/progestin combinations such as CombiPatch and FemHRT
- Micronized oral progesterone, marketed as Prometrium

Progestin can be taken continuously, cyclically (twelve to fourteen days of every month), or in a pulsed regimen of three days on and three days off. Progestins given in a cyclic fashion usually produce a predictable menstrual period; progestins given in the same dose on a daily basis are designed to make most women amenorrheic, or period-free, after one year of therapy or sooner.

ALERT

Your health care professional can adjust your hormone prescription or use as necessary. Since the progestin works to prevent endometrial cancer, don't experiment with your progestin dosage or the number of days that you take it each month, without consulting your physician.

Androgens in HRT

Androgens are male hormones that are normally produced in small quantities by the ovaries and adrenal glands, with the greatest quantities occurring at the midpoint of a woman's cycle. Androgens contribute to bone density (though not as dramatically as do estrogens), and some studies show that they might promote a healthy libido by fostering a desire for sex. Androgen production also drops dramatically when ovarian function decreases around the time of perimenopause. The decrease is even more dramatic if a woman undergoes a surgical menopause. If women have severe menopausal or perimenopausal symptoms such as intermittent hot flashes or a greatly reduced sex drive, despite a trial of traditional HRT, their health care providers may recommend an HRT regimen that includes androgens.

The use of androgens to combat menopausal symptoms is relatively new, unlike estrogen, which has been used and studied since the mid-1950s. Some studies have shown that androgen in combination with estrogen not only slows bone loss but also may help promote the growth of new bone tissue. Some experts believe androgens help alleviate other menopausal symptoms such as hot flashes and vaginal dryness. Androgens carry some negative risks, of course; some studies suggest that androgen can have a negative effect on blood cholesterol levels, and a few patients who take androgens can experience unwanted side effects, such as the growth of excess body hair (especially on the face), acne, or oiliness of the skin. In general, androgens are added to an HRT regimen only if libido or hot flashes are not improved on standard HRT dosages.

FACTS

Long-term studies are essential for understanding the full implications of any drug or medical treatment. The National Institutes of Health's Women's Health Initiative Study is a fifteen-year study launched in 1991 to study the most common causes of death, disability, and diminished quality of life in postmenopausal women, including a representative sample of them who used HRT, and another group taking estrogen alone.

The Facts about HRT

Perimenopausal and postmenopausal women have a variety of alternatives for protecting their health and diminishing menopausal symptoms. The most popular and proven of these is hormone replacement therapy. However, many women are reluctant to begin HRT, and many women who start HRT discontinue it within six months. HRT isn't for everyone. Your family or personal medical history may make you a poor candidate for hormone replacement therapy. Or you may choose to use other methods for maintaining your health and alleviating menopausal symptoms. However, your choice should be based on fact—not unnecessary fears or unfounded beliefs about the safety or beneficial impact of this treatment option. This section presents those facts.

Unfortunately, much of the information available to the public about HRT is wrong or misleading—based on questionable science and unscientific studies. Some media seem dedicated to promoting only controversial or negative findings regarding health care issues and the medical establishment, in order to fan the public's fear (and boost ratings). Your trained, licensed health care provider is your best source of complete information and advice about HRT, how it works, and what risks and benefits it offers you.

When you're considering hormone replacement therapy, talk with your health care provider, ask questions, explore alternatives, and get a second opinion. If you need to consult with several health care professionals—do it! And check Appendix B, Resources, for a list of useful, solid sources of medical information.

Who Uses HRT?

Hormone replacement therapy is used by fewer than half of all menopausal women in the United States. The reasons for using—or not using—HRT vary from individual to individual, but many women who aren't on HRT have yet to make a decision regarding its use. The decision to follow an HRT regimen is an important one for any woman;

as soon as your ovarian function diminishes, your hormone levels plummet. Whatever technique you use to minimize postmenopausal bone loss, heart disease, muscle and other tissue degradation, memory function loss, and other effects of diminished hormones, you need to begin it before those losses build. Here's what we know about the women who choose HRT and why they choose it:

- Though findings vary, most surveys indicate that the main reason women between the ages of fifty and fifty-five choose to begin HRT is for the relief of hot flashes and other vasomotor symptoms. Women who begin HRT at age sixty-five and older are more likely to be concerned with preventing or postponing the onset of osteoporosis.
- Almost 40 percent of perimenopausal women turn to HRT for the relief of night sweats and vaginal dryness—in addition to hot flashes.
- A 1997 survey reported in the *Journal of Women's Health* discovered that nearly fifty percent of those who were currently using HRT had undergone a hysterectomy. In that study, over 35 percent of current HRT users and over 40 percent of past users turned to HRT as a result of surgically induced menopause. Understandably, women who no longer have a uterus have little concern over irregular vaginal bleeding.

The Benefits of HRT

HRT offers women a number of sound, solid health benefits—both in the relief of symptoms and in the prevention of some serious health threats that result from the body's loss of hormones after their ovaries cease to function.

Don't overlook the importance of getting a bone density screening test! Osteopenia—early bone loss not severe enough to qualify as osteoporosis but a definite warning sign—is present in over two-thirds of the population of women. These statistics have emerged only recently, as bone density screening tests have become more common.

HRT has proven its benefit in maintaining bone health and preventing osteoporosis. Osteoporosis threatens nearly 28 million Americans—and 80 percent of those threatened are women. Nearly 30 percent of all women over age sixty-five have osteoporosis, and many of them don't know it until symptoms become painfully obvious, as happens when a bone crumbles or snaps. Most studies show that women who use estrogen and progestin HRT compounds reduce their risk of hip fracture by 11 percent for each year of HRT treatments. Here are just some of the other benefits of hormone replacement therapy:

- HRT is the most time-proven methods for mitigating hot flashes, vaginal dryness, and other uncomfortable menopausal symptoms.
- Estrogen may help protect memory functions by improving circulation and increasing the flow of nourishing blood to the brain; early studies seem to indicate that it may help delay or prevent the onset of Alzheimer's disease.
- Estrogen may be effective in protecting the health of the eyes, postponing or preventing the onset of macular degeneration—the leading cause of blindness in those age sixty-five and older. Macular degeneration is the most common cause of failures for the eye examination required in the driver's license recertification process. A lack of the ability to drive a car is one of the most common causes of loss of independence and feelings of isolation and depression among the elderly.
- Estrogen reduces the risk of contracting colorectal cancer by as much as a third in most studies.

FACTS

Macular degeneration often takes the form of a clouding of the eye's lens. Age-related macular degeneration (AMD) causes the retina to deteriorate, and it's usually noticeable first as a clouding of the central area of vision (the peripheral vision can remain intact). AMD is the leading cause of night blindness in the United States. Many doctors recommend HRT to prevent or control the onset of AMD.

The Risks of HRT

If you read the newspaper, listen to the evening news, or pick up any women's magazine, you're likely to read or hear about ongoing research into the risks and benefits of HRT almost daily. Because HRT has been under study for so long, some reports about its potential risks are inevitable, but further study is needed to understand fully its long-term effects. Any medication carries certain risks. Here are the HRT risks most women must consider:

Breast cancer: A small number of recent studies suggest that long-term (more than five years) estrogen use in HRT may result in a small but increased risk of breast cancer. Though this risk appears to be small, most health care professionals advise women who have a personal history of breast cancer against using HRT for at least the first five years following their diagnoses. A family history of breast cancer in an aunt on your father's side doesn't have the same impact on your health history as does an occurrence of breast cancer in your mother or sister—considered first-degree relatives. Regardless of their use of HRT or family history, all menopausal women should get regular mammograms, conduct monthly self-breast exams, and visit their physician annually.

Endometrial cancer: If you still have your uterus, you shouldn't take unopposed estrogen (estrogen without progesterone) for the sole purpose of relief of menopausal symptoms, because unopposed estrogen can increase your risk of developing endometrial cancer. HRT programs that balance estrogen with progestin eliminate this risk, however, and may in fact help reduce the risk of endometrial cancer even further compared to women who take no hormone supplements. If you have been treated successfully for early (Stage I through III) endometrial cancer, with a total hysterectomy, your doctor may recommend an ERT regimen for you after a certain disease-free interval, usually three to five years.

Blood clots: If you have ever developed blood clots in the deep veins of your legs or in your lungs or eyes, you may be susceptible to redeveloping them if you use HRT. High levels of estrogen can contribute to this condition, so your health care professional will want to test your current blood hormone levels and review your history to see if you are a good candidate for HRT. Low-dose estrogen treatments may not complicate your risks for recurring blood clots, so your doctor may recommend that HRT option. Your doctor can order special blood tests that check for clotting difficulties, if your family or personal medical history raises any question about an inherited susceptibility.

Irregular bleeding or spotting is the most common side effect complaint of women on HRT, while others report breast tenderness and water retention. And, while some women say HRT contributes to migraines, others say it actually helps ameliorate migraine problems they've experienced for years.

Liver disease: If you have active liver disease or if your liver's functions have become seriously impaired through illness or injury, you aren't a good candidate for HRT. Your liver is the organ that metabolizes (breaks down) the estrogen in your circulatory system. If your liver isn't functioning properly, your body won't be able to metabolize the estrogen component of HRT. If your liver disease is resolved, however, the threat of this potential for an increased risk may have passed. Your doctor or health care professional can advise you whether your liver function (usually based on blood tests for liver enzymes) makes you a good candidate for HRT.

The increased risk of breast cancer is slight; most studies indicate that among women who took estrogen for five years, HRT contributed to only one additional case of breast cancer in every 1,000 women. The overall risk of breast cancer for women age sixty to sixty-five who aren't taking estrogen is low—about 350 of every 100,000 women on average. That number rises to 400 of every 100,000 for women of the same age who take estrogen. Regular mammograms are the key to proper monitoring. HRT may not play as beneficial a role in protecting women against heart disease as was once thought. Partial results of the Women's Health Initiative study, released in July 2002, revealed a slight increase in nonfatal heart attack, stroke, and pulmonary embolus in women taking HRT, as compared to women taking placebo alone. That portion of the study is ongoing.

When the final, complete results of the long-term Women's Health Initiative are gathered (in 2005), the medical and scientific communities will have a much clearer understanding of the long-term benefits and risks of HRT. Until then, discuss all of your options, concerns, and questions with your health care provider, and make an informed decision. Don't let unspecified fears or suspicions stop you in your tracks when you're preparing a health plan for this important phase of your adult life.

HRT Options

Because HRT is such a widely used and studied method of treatment, a number of different HRT compounds and delivery methods have developed over the years. You and your doctor can determine the form that's best for you, but here are some of the most popular options:

- Pills can offer estrogen or estrogen/progestin combinations that are taken continuously, cyclically, or in pulse patterns of, for example, three days on then three days off.
- Patches can deliver a steady dose of estrogen or estrogen/progestin combinations every day of the month. You change patches every three to seven days, and you can wear them when swimming or showering.
- Flexible vaginal rings deliver estrogen in steady doses to women who suffer from vaginal dryness. Some forms are available that make estrogen replacement safe even for breast cancer patients, because the estrogen works locally (in the vagina), and is not absorbed into the bloodstream (which could increase the potential for the recurrence of the cancer).
- Creams and gels provide topical estrogen or progesterone doses to women who suffer from vaginal dryness. Both creams and gels are applied directly inside the vagina; some women rub vaginal progesterone gels and creams directly on the skin. Again, your health care provider can advise you on the proper dose and delivery mechanism for these (and all) forms of HRT.

Not all hormone creams and gels are approved by the FDA (Food and Drug Administration). Be sure to consult your physician regarding proper dosage, possible side effects, and application of these creams.

A new option, called low-dose HRT, has shown promising results in a number of studies, including that reported by Dr. Bruce Ettinger in the August, 2001 issue of *Journal of Obstetrics and Gynecology*. In that study, 138 women between the ages of fifty-five and seventy-five who had been using standard doses of HRT (.625 mg of conjugated estrogen with monthly doses of a type of progestin called MPA) were switched to 0.3 mg of estrogen daily with fourteen-day programs of MPA administered every six months. The study indicated that the reduced levels of hormones were effective in reducing symptoms and caused very little vaginal bleeding—one of the primary objections many women express to traditional HRT. The protection against osteoporosis conferred by the lower dose is nearly the same as that seen with the standard dose.

It is anticipated that the future trend in HRT will be toward the use of the lowest possible doses that can treat vasomotor symptoms and still reduce a woman's risk for bone fractures. Talk with your doctor or health care provider for more details.

Designer Estrogens

In the past several years, a number of artificial estrogens have been developed to provide some of the benefits of estrogen replacement therapy while avoiding some of the risks for women who aren't good candidates for HRT. In other words, the artificial estrogens act like estrogens with some of the body's tissues, but they don't act like estrogens with others. These so-called "designer estrogens" are more correctly referred to as selective estrogen receptor modulators or SERMs. Some health care providers prescribe SERMs to combat bone loss in postmenopausal patients who can't or choose not to use HRT, but who are at risk of developing osteoporosis. Following are the most common SERMs in use today.

- Tamoxifen (sold under the brand name Nolvadex) has been in use for some years to help reduce the potential for recurrence of estrogen-dependent breast cancer in women with a history of that disease. Ongoing study and scrutiny of Tamoxifen indicate that it isn't an "ideal answer" for postmenopausal women. Some studies have linked it to an increased risk of endometrial polyps, blood clots, and possibly precancerous endometrial hyperplasia.

- Raloxifene was approved by the FDA in 1997 for use in the prevention of osteoporosis, and was marketed in 1998 under the brand name Evista. Though still under study, raloxifene has been found to maintain a certain amount of bone density, at least in some patients, without increasing the risk of breast or uterine cancer. Because it doesn't appear to have any adverse effects on the endometrium, women who still have their uterus don't need to take progestin or progesterone when on raloxifene. However, some studies show that raloxifene is only about half as effective as estrogen at increasing bone density. Raloxifene's effect on cholesterol is still unknown; though it appears to reduce LDL cholesterol, it hasn't been shown to increase "good" HDL cholesterol the way estrogen does. The risk of blood clots with raloxifene seems to be similar to that of estrogen, and raloxifene has shown no beneficial effect in reducing hot flashes. It actually increases hot flashes in some patients.

Though SERMs show great promise for the development of postmenopausal treatment without the risks of traditional hormones, none of the SERMs has been around long enough to have passed scrutiny in long-term use studies. Newer SERMs with fewer side effects are in development.

Weighing Risks and Benefits

So how do you decide whether to use HRT or what form of HRT is best for you? You've probably guessed the answer to this one—talk with your doctor or health care professional. Reading this book and studying the other resources it mentions (see Appendix B for a list of published and online resources) is an important step toward educating yourself about the risks and benefits of HRT, but you always benefit from a professional's firsthand experience and advice when making this decision. When you meet with your health care professional, ask about the following tests and risks factors:

- Talk to your doctor about your personal and family history of osteoporosis, heart disease, breast cancer, blood clots, colon cancer, and liver disease.
- Ask about a bone density test to determine the current state of your bone health. A heel or peripheral bone density test may give you all the information you need, and is cheaper and quicker to perform than some more detailed bone examinations. It is especially appropriate the first time you are screened for osteoporosis.
- Request a fasting blood test called a "lipid profile" to find out your levels of total cholesterol, HDL, LDL, and triglycerides to determine your cardiac disease risk.
- Ask your doctor about the usefulness of blood tests to determine your current blood hormone levels, or how close you are to menopause.
- Keep your menstrual journal or menstrual symptom diary (see "The Journey Through Perimenopause" in Chapter 3) and take it with you to discuss the symptoms you've been having and their severity, so you know what kind of symptom relief you need most.
- Ask your doctor or health care professional about alternatives to HRT, their benefits, and their drawbacks.

Part of a Healthy Menopause Plan

Hormone replacement therapy offers an enormous number of benefits for women in perimenopause, menopause, and postmenopause. But lifestyle and behavioral changes are an important part of a complete plan for a healthy life—before, during, and after the onset of menopause. No pill, patch, or cream will keep you healthy if you live an unhealthy lifestyle. As you grow older, your health maintenance becomes more critical—and more demanding. So even if you adopt a full program of HRT—or use any HRT alternative—you need to follow the guidelines listed below to maintain your good health:

- Eat a healthy diet that's high in vegetables, fruits, and whole grains, and low in saturated fat and red meat. If you're interested in maintaining strong muscles, healthy bones, and good heart health, your first priority must be a good diet.
- Get plenty of exercise. Weight-bearing exercise, such as walking or weight lifting, improves the health of your heart, develops muscle mass, reduces body fat, and builds strong bones. The best HRT program in the world won't protect your health if you turn into a couch potato.
- Get plenty of sleep. Sleep deprivation contributes to anxiety, depression, and fatigue—the most troublesome symptoms of hormone depletion.
- Stop smoking. Smoking not only harms your health but also increases your risk for certain types of cancers that are more common in menopause. Smoking and estrogen are a bad combination; do yourself and everyone who loves you a favor, and kick the habit. You can do it; visit the American Cancer Society at ✎ *www.cancer.org*, and search for "Preparing to Quit," for help in finding a number of proven tactics, or ask your health care provider for suggestions.
- Get regular medical checkups. Your doctor will recommend annual examinations to monitor the progress of your HRT program. During the exam, your health care provider will check your breasts for lumps; do a pelvic exam to determine the health of your uterus, cervix, vagina, and ovaries; and check your blood pressure. Don't skip these appointments; they're an important part of your HRT program. Ask about screening for colon cancer as well.

Remember to follow your HRT program exactly as prescribed. Many people forget their schedule, and miss doses. Use whatever reminder mechanism works for you—a weekly pill container, a marked calendar, notes on your mirror, or other device. If you can't find a reminder that works, ask your health care professional for advice. But don't miss doses!

CHAPTER 12
Alternatives to HRT

Hormone replacement therapy isn't the answer for every woman's desire for symptom relief. Many women choose not to use traditional HRT, and others aren't suitable candidates for HRT as a result of a personal or family medical history. If you are among these women—or are simply interested in learning more about nonhormonal treatment options—this chapter provides some good information about HRT alternatives.

Why Some Women Choose HRT Alternatives

Chapter 11, "Understanding Hormones and HRT," presented some reasons for choosing an alternative to HRT for combating the symptoms and health-threatening physical changes of menopause. Doctors and health care professionals may discourage women who have personal medical histories of deep vein blood clots, active liver disease, and breast cancer, for example, from using HRT. If these women were to take regular doses of estrogen and cyclic doses of progesterone, they could suffer a complication or, in rare cases, a recurrence of their prior medical condition.

FACTS

Don't count on conventional wisdom to guide you in choosing HRT or an alternative. The potential for complications resulting from estrogen and/or progesterone use differs from individual to individual, depending on dosage and personal medical history. Your doctor or health care provider can best advise you on this issue.

Placing Emphasis on Choice

Medical complications aren't the only factor that might send a woman in search of an alternative to HRT. Some of the reasons women cite for choosing not to use traditional hormone replacement therapies follow:

Troublesome side effects of HRT: Many women who begin HRT later discontinue its use, citing progestin-related side effects, including vaginal bleeding, breast tenderness, bloating, depression, and irritability, as conditions that discouraged them from continuing the treatment. New progestins are now available that differ dramatically from those previously available, so don't forget to discuss new pharmaceutical treatment options with your doctor.

Fear of an increased risk of cancer: Many women fear that estrogen or other hormones included in traditional HRT regimens will increase their risk of cancer, even when they have no personal or family medical history of the disease.

Aversion to the "medicalization" of a natural process: A 1997 survey conducted by the North American Menopause Society found that nearly half of American women surveyed considered menopause a natural process that doesn't require medical management.

Do sound medical statistics support these reasons? Most studies indicate that HRT is safe and effective for most perimenopausal and menopausal women. Many women who experience side effects while on HRT find that after a period of a few months those symptoms lessen or disappear entirely. No responsible medical authority would encourage a woman with a medical history that puts her at an increased risk for developing (or redeveloping) cancer or other diseases and illness to take HRT. A calm, thorough discussion with your health care provider (and getting a second opinion) is the best method for assessing the potential risks and rewards of HRT for you.

The "medicalization" question is one each woman must decide for herself. Only you can decide whether the potential benefits of HRT outweigh your resistance to replacing your body's naturally diminishing hormones. But take time to really assess your position on this issue; every time you take an aspirin to relieve a headache or use an antibiotic ointment to protect a cut or scratch, you're altering very natural processes. And if you begin a regimen of any herb, pharmaceutical, or supplement to offset the symptoms and physical changes of menopause, you are attempting to manage the process.

Alternative therapies aren't inexpensive. A recent survey found that the average vitamin/mineral/nutritional menopause symptom treatment costs about $2.00 per tablet—essentially the same as the cost of the usual dose of HRT. If cost is your only problem, investigate some prescription drug discount programs or seek out Internet pharmacies—the cost, especially if you purchase in bulk (usually three months supplies), is at least one-fourth to one-third less than that at your standard pharmacy.

No one right or wrong answer applies to every woman. Each individual must educate herself about all treatment options, then work closely with a trusted health care professional to make this highly personal choice. Remember, this isn't your mother's menopause. Your mother didn't have the advantages of the scientific advancements in the treatment of menopausal symptoms and the wide range of preventative medications to ward off debilitating diseases such as osteoporosis. You have a wealth of information and options available to you for managing your health through menopause. Take advantage of the benefits of scientific advancements and research that are available for improving the quality of your life.

FACTS

Although only a few studies out of thousands have shown a slightly increased risk of breast cancer following long-term use (ten or more years) of HRT, most medical authorities agree that short-term use of estrogen/progestin combination HRT (fewer than five years) does not lead to an increased risk of developing breast cancer. See Chapter 11 for more information on this topic.

Of course, many other reasons may be a factor in discouraging women from using HRT. Many women haven't the funds for ongoing medical therapy and are uninsured or underinsured, and therefore, can't afford it. These women face multiple challenges in finding affordable alternatives to HRT, since many insurance programs refuse to cover certain alternative treatments. Some women may choose to avoid any kind of medical treatment as a result of religious or philosophical beliefs. For these women, nonmedical alternatives to HRT offer the only options for maintaining physical and emotional health during the transition through menopause.

Remembering the Medical Impact of Menopause

When you're weighing the pros and cons of choosing HRT or an alternative, it's important to remember that you have much more to be concerned about than the physical discomforts of hot flashes or occasional forgetfulness and mood swings. Your body's lack of estrogen can lead to real problems such as osteoporosis and vaginal atrophy. Avoiding HRT doesn't automatically make you a natural woman or a stronger, more capable individual. If anything, it may leave you less able by exposing you to multiple health problems associated with aging.

If you choose not to take HRT for either medical or personal reasons, you need to adopt other means of protecting your bones, brain, skin, and heart as you age. As you consider alternatives to HRT, it's important that you remember the full range of symptoms and conditions you may need to combat. Some of the most common symptoms of perimenopause and menopause are:

- Hot flashes
- Mood swings
- Decreased sexual drive
- Difficulty concentrating
- Heart palpitations
- Migraine headaches
- Irregular and/or heavy periods
- Involuntary urine release and bladder urgency
- Insomnia
- Panic attacks

Some of the health issues that women face as they age and their natural hormone production diminishes dramatically in menopause are:

- Heart disease
- High blood pressure
- Cholesterol imbalances
- Osteoporosis
- Loss of muscle mass
- Vision problems related to macular degeneration
- Decreased cognitive functions

- Joint disease
- Urinary tract disorders
- Vaginal dryness and painful intercourse
- Weight gain

Will any one treatment program combat all of these symptoms and conditions? No, it's unlikely that any single alternative treatment option will be able to solve all of the physical problems and symptoms of hormone loss and aging. That's why any treatment option you choose must be part of a balanced, lifelong program of healthy living and careful health management. Diet, exercise, regular medical checkups, and an active, engaged lifestyle are critical to preserving your ongoing health—through menopause and beyond.

ALERT

Don't look to any one source—especially popular consumer magazines or chat rooms on the Internet—for information about menopause. Reading this book is a good start; check the Resources section (Appendix B) for other sources of sound information. Talk to your health care provider and other health care professionals to get second—even third—opinions.

Nonhormonal Medications

Many women use nonhormonal medications to combat the initial symptoms of menopause, including hot flashes, insomnia, sexual dysfunction, depression, mood swings, and fatigue. Medical treatments and preventatives for some physical conditions such as cholesterol imbalances, high blood pressure, bone loss, and vaginal dryness also are available. Only your doctor or health care professional can determine whether you are a good candidate for any or all of these pharmaceuticals, but this section offers a brief overview of some of the most widely prescribed and effective nonhormonal medications in use for the treatment of menopause symptoms.

For Hot Flashes and Night Sweats

Hot flashes are the perimenopausal and menopausal symptom many women report as the most bothersome. Hot flashes and night sweats are types of vasomotor symptoms some women experience as their natural hormone production slows then stops in the years preceding and following menopause. Hot flashes can be mild flushes that spread across the face and neck and pass quickly, or they can be debilitating waves of increased skin temperature that can last up to thirty minutes and leave a woman drenched in sweat and exhausted from the experience. Night sweats can interrupt sleep or cause insomnia, and lead to fatigue, exhaustion, and a diminished attention span and cognitive function. In other words, vasomotor symptoms aren't minor inconveniences for many women—they're serious conditions with both physical and emotional side effects.

Although estrogen is considered by many doctors to be the best choice for the relief of vasomotor symptoms associated with menopause, some other medications are available to diminish their impact. Progestin, progesterone compounds, and progesterone creams have shown some effectiveness in reducing the frequency and severity of hot flashes, as have low doses of clonidine and methyldopa, medications traditionally used in the treatment of high blood pressure. Some studies indicate that some antidepressants, for example, venlafaxine hydrochloride (marketed under the name Effexor), prescribed in very low doses, may offer some relief from vasomotor symptoms. (See Chapter 16 for information about pharmaceutical and alternative treatments.)

FACTS

Many women who have a personal history of breast cancer turn to nonhormonal medications for the control of hot flashes and night sweats. Ongoing research continues to refine the medical world's knowledge of these drugs and their impact on vasomotor symptoms. Your doctor or health care professional must prescribe any pharmaceutical, and is your best source for information regarding these medications.

Though each of these drug types offers both benefits and potential negative side effects, one of them may be a good treatment alternative for your menopausal hot flashes and night sweats. New medical treatments for hot flashes emerge daily.

For Blood Pressure and Cholesterol Management

Estrogen replacement has been shown to be an effective tool for normalizing cholesterol levels in women as they pass through menopause. Normal levels of estrogen help to raise "good" HDL cholesterol and lower "bad" LDL cholesterol. Estrogen also helps keep the arterial walls flexible, clean, and wide; as your natural estrogen diminishes, your chances of developing high blood pressure increase. Though diet and exercise are your two most effective means for controlling cholesterol levels and blood pressure, many medications are currently available to treat both conditions:

- Simvastatin, Pravastatin, and Lovastatin are just some of the cholesterol-controlling drugs that fall within a category known as HMG-CoA reductase inhibitors. Drugs in this category work by blocking an enzyme that your body uses to produce cholesterol, so they have been shown to be very effective in lowering cholesterol levels and preventing deaths due to heart disease. These drugs can interact with some other medications, and they aren't often recommended for people with active liver disease.
- Diuretics flush water and sodium from the body and can be effective for reducing blood pressure. Diuretic drugs include thiazides, potassium-sparing diuretics, and loop diuretics. You may have heard these drugs referred to as "water pills," but they're much more powerful than that name would imply. Diuretics reduce the level of fluid in your bloodstream and help remove sodium from your circulation, so they may help open up arteries and boost the capacity of your arterial system and thereby lower blood pressure against your arterial walls. However, if you do not have high blood pressure and don't have a tendency to retain water, they may not be appropriate for you.
- Beta blockers, including lopranonol and metroprolol, block some of the nerve impulses to the heart; as a result, the heartbeat slows and

the heart's workload decreases. Doctors often prescribe beta blockers along with diuretics to control blood pressure. Sometimes beta blockers are combined with alpha blockers—drugs that relax blood vessels—in one medication called an alpha-beta blocker. Labetalol is one example of these alpha-beta blocking drugs. All of these medications are extremely powerful, and therefore are carefully prescribed and monitored by doctors and other medical professionals.

- ACE inhibitors are also effective in controlling high blood pressure, and they seem to work by inhibiting the formation of the hormone angiotensin II—a substance that causes blood vessels to constrict. Researchers are still trying to determine exactly how these drugs work to lower blood pressure, but some doctors are prescribing them for that purpose.

High blood pressure medications have a range of possible side effects, and most doctors recommend other methods as a first line of defense against this disease. Controlling dietary fat, salt intake, and (of course) stopping smoking are the most effective weapons against high blood pressure. But for some women, medication is a necessary component of their plan for combating hypertension.

If you have access to the Internet, you can turn to the National Institutes of Health's National Medical Library for authoritative information about most drugs prescribed today. Use the Library's topic list, drug information, and dictionaries to find out how any drug works, how it's prescribed, and its potential side effects and interactions. Find the library at ✐*www.nlm.nih.gov* (click on MEDLINEplus).

For Managing Bone Loss

Though estrogen is the undisputed queen of bone maintenance, medical science has made a number of strides in finding alternative drugs for slowing the bone deterioration associated with the estrogen deficiency of menopause. Weight-bearing exercise and a diet rich in calcium and vitamin D are important components of any plan to maintain good bone health. (See Chapter 8 for more information.) The following medications are other options for preventing or slowing the progress of osteoporosis:

Alendronate: an FDA-approved biphosphonate that helps slow the breakdown of bone tissue that occurs in osteoporosis. According to the American College of Obstetrics and Gynecology, some research trials on this drug have shown that it not only helps slow bone loss but also may even build bone tissue in the spine and hip—two areas most prone to the complications of osteoporosis and possible fracture. Alendronate has been associated with irritation of the esophagus in a small percentage of patients, but new dosages and formulations are under development that will reduce its potential for negative side effects. A new once-a-week dosage significantly reduces short-term side effects.

Risedronate: a drug that inhibits the body's ability to reabsorb bone tissue, and thereby slows bone loss. The FDA approved this drug in 2000. Risedronate doesn't seem to cause as much stomach or esophageal irritation as alendronate. It also protects the bone density of the total body and reduces the risk of fracture in the spinal vertebrae and the hip, especially in high-risk women.

Calcitonin: not really a nonhormonal treatment for osteoporosis but a hormone produced by the parathyroid gland, calcitonin is available as a prescription drug. Calcitonin helps slow bone loss by slowing bone resorption, in a process similar to the previous two drugs in this list. Typically, calcitonin is given as a nasal spray that you take two times a day. It has been shown to be useful in reducing the risk of fractures of the spinal vertebrae in very elderly women; it does not lessen the risk of hip fracture or protect younger women.

Another drug that doesn't quite fit the description of a nonhormonal approach to fighting osteoporosis is raloxifene—an artificial hormone used as an alternative to estrogen. Raloxifene was approved by the FDA in 1997 for the prevention of osteoporosis, and studies have shown that it maintains bone density in some women (though not quite as well as estrogen) and may prevent fractures of the spine, but not the hip. Raloxifene may cause hot flashes, and though it lowers LDL cholesterol it doesn't raise HDL cholesterol. It is not considered as beneficial as estrogen for the bone or the heart. (See Chapter 11 for more details.)

For Combating Insomnia, Depression, and Anxiety

Though thousands of people in the United States suffer from sleep disorders, insomnia becomes a true enemy of women as they approach menopause. Hormonal fluctuations lead to night sweats and mini panic attacks that can blast a woman out of a sound sleep at three A.M. and keep her awake for hours. Sleep disturbances are integrally linked with depression and anxiety. Insomnia is also linked to high blood pressure, fatigue, and a long list of other physical and emotional disorders.

SSENTIALS

The National Sleep Foundation recommends that any type of sleep-aiding medication be used only in conjunction with lifestyle changes, including diet restrictions, exercise, a regular sleep schedule, and a managed sleep environment. Even then, the NSF recommends that use of the sleep aids be short-term or intermittent.

Lifestyle changes are essential to guarding your sleep and leading a calm, rested—and energetic—life. Exercise, stress-management techniques, and a diet low in caffeine and alcohol all are important components of any plan to maintain deep, restful sleep and emotional health. Though many doctors recommend HRT for the relief of insomnia, depression, and anxiety, a number of medications are available to help menopausal women combat these debilitating conditions.

Hypnotics, also known as benzodiazepine agonists, have been used to treat insomnia since the 1960s. These drugs, including triazolam, zolpidem, and zaleplon, promote falling asleep and remaining asleep throughout the night. These drugs are considered relatively risk-free, but most doctors recommend using them only for short-term treatment. Because hypnotics affect the brain's activity for a short period during the night, they can cause a loss of balance and falls in people who get up to use the restroom during the night (not uncommon during perimenopause and menopause). The drug may also have a residual effect upon awakening, making you feel tired and sluggish when you try to get up.

Antidepressants can provide true relief from the symptoms of major depression that some women report during perimenopause and menopause. The variety and effectiveness of antidepressants have increased tremendously in the past two decades, and the development of a new generation of medications in this class, SSRIs, has broadened the applications of their use to make them more practical for many who suffer depression. Because SSRIs, such as fluoxetine and sertraline, don't make the body produce more serotonin, but simply make better use of its existing levels, these drugs are not addictive and don't result in an artificial high of good feeling. Your doctor or health care professional will work closely with you to determine whether you are a good candidate for antidepressants and which will work best for you.

If you have sleep apnea or have to operate heavy machinery soon after awakening, your doctor is unlikely to recommend hypnotics as treatment for insomnia. Hypnotics can actually make breathing even more difficult for those with sleep apnea, and some hypnotics can continue having an impact on brain functions long enough to impair your abilities shortly after awakening.

Anxiolytics, such as buspirone and alprazolam, are antianxiety drugs that many health care professionals prescribe to lessen the effects of depression, anxiety, and sleeplessness in perimenopausal and menopausal women. Anxiolytics also can treat the symptoms of premenstrual dysphoric disorder (PMDD) that many perimenopausal women experience as they move closer to menopause. These drugs can have a slightly sedative effect, so many health care professionals prescribe them only for short periods of time, especially for the treatment of PMDD (when they may be prescribed for just the week or ten to fourteen days preceding the onset of menstrual flow).

Prescription medications can offer true relief from many of the symptoms and physical conditions that result from perimenopause and menopause. But they aren't your only—and many times not even the best—answer. HRT effectively combats many of these conditions, but your lifestyle choices are always the first tool you should turn to for maintaining your health and emotional well-being at any stage of life. The following sections discuss supplemental vitamins and nutrients and a range of therapeutic programs that can also help keep you strong, fit, and healthy through menopause.

There's a big difference between major depression and a generalized, intermittent feeling of the "blues." Most health care professionals recommend lifestyle adjustments as the first-line defense against these and other emotional disorders. See Chapter 10 for more information.

Herbs, Plant Estrogens, and Supplements

Women have been using herbs to combat the symptoms of menopause for centuries—in fact, only in the past century have any other options been available. As pharmaceutical science has evolved over the past hundred years, so has our understanding of the benefits of supplementing a healthy diet with vitamin and mineral compounds. Today, nearly every woman takes some form of vitamin, herb, or nutritional supplement at some time—if not throughout her life. Most health care experts recommend that women supplement a healthy diet with certain vitamins and minerals as they approach menopause.

As a woman's body begins changing with the approach of menopause, its nutritional needs change. And the effects of hormonal imbalance and depletion present special problems that many women choose to address with a nonpharmaceutical solution. Many women turn to botanical compounds, plant and herb extracts, and nutritional supplements to alleviate the symptoms of perimenopause and to offset the physical changes the body can experience as a result of estrogen depletion and the natural aging process.

Plant substances aren't inherently safer or more benign than laboratory produced chemicals, but they're not subject to FDA approval. Plant extracts can be very powerful and can interact with prescription or nonprescription drugs to cause dangerous side effects. Don't take any substance without fully understanding its effects, and ask your health care provider if it's safe for you.

Choosing Natural Alternatives Wisely

You can't walk down the aisle of any grocery, pharmacy, or health food store without finding an ever-growing selection of herbal compounds and other botanical treatments that offer a natural approach to better health. An increasing number of botanical supplements are available for the management of menopausal symptoms. Some of these alternatives are effective— some aren't. Some of them can be downright dangerous when taken without the knowledge or advice of a trained nutritionist or health care professional. Because the sale of herbal compounds and nutraceuticals— foods that also deliver some sort of medication or compound designed to offer a specific medical benefit—has become such big business, it has drawn the attention of the popular media as well as the medical community.

Frequent articles in magazines, newspapers, and on Internet pages discuss the latest vitamin or herbal alternatives, and the scientific community continues to test and release results on the efficacy of these compounds for the treatment of specific physical or emotional disorders. Because botanical extracts and nutritional supplements aren't subject to FDA approval, each consumer is responsible for making the wisest, most informed choice when buying these products. The need for information for women seeking a natural alternative to HRT for the relief of menopausal symptoms is especially critical; the alternatives must offer relief from a range of overt symptoms while, at the same time, supplementing the body's supply of important vitamins and minerals.

Consider the following important points when you're assessing the value of choosing herbs and/or nutritional supplements for the treatment of menopausal symptoms:

Are you looking for symptom relief or health maintenance? Many herbal alternatives are effective for relieving a single symptom or for supplementing a specific nutritional need. The wider the range of relief you are seeking, the more pills, capsules, powders, and teas you may need to consume. And you will need your health care professional to assess the safety of that combination.

Have you already adopted the healthy lifestyle changes recommended for women at your stage of life? A proper diet, regular exercise, and good stress-management skills are as essential for those using alternative treatments for menopausal symptoms as they are for women using HRT. No botanical compound, vitamin collection, or nutritional supplement will replace these very basic necessities for maintaining your health through menopause.

Have you talked with others who are using the treatment alternative you're considering, and have you discussed it with your health care provider? Making a decision to use these alternatives requires that you educate yourself on all of the possible benefits and drawbacks of your choice. Again, don't think you can tinker with harmless experimentation. Your choice of botanical and nutritional supplements that are powerful enough to treat the symptoms and diminish the physical degradation of bone, muscle, and brain tissue that accompanies menopause requires your careful consideration and thorough research.

FACTS

No alternative medication or herb can surpass the results of modern scientific technology and the pharmaceuticals it has provided us. When deciding on a plan to maintain your long-term health during and after menopause, get the authoritative information and advice you need to make an intelligent decision.

The range of botanical substances, nutritional supplements, and nutraceuticals available for perimenopausal and menopausal women is vast. Appendix B contains a number of authoritative references for more information on this topic. The following sections list some of the most popular—and promising—herbs, plant extracts, and nutritional supplements in use today for management of menopausal symptoms.

QUESTIONS?

What is a bioflavonoid?
Bioflavonoids are naturally occurring plant substances found in many brightly colored fruits and vegetables, such as cherries, oranges and other citrus, grapes, leafy vegetables, wine, and some types of red clover. Researchers are studying bioflavonoids for the treatment of a number of conditions, including the control of bleeding, hemorrhoids, and varicose veins.

Understanding Plant Hormones

So how can a plant or herb compound relieve the symptoms of hormone depletion and imbalance? The answer to that question lies in the chemical makeup of certain plants that contain phytohormones—natural substances found in some herbs and other plants that may help to regulate the plant's growth. Though plant and human hormones are very different substances, phytohormones (some types are referred to as phytoestrogens) can bind to the human body's estrogen receptors; phytoestrogens may act like an estrogen on the body or like an antiestrogen, depending upon their particular type and dosage.

Two of the most popular types of phytoestrogens used in menopausal supplements today are isoflavones (a class of bioflavonoids) and lignans. Isoflavones occur in soybeans, red clover, and (in much lower quantities) green tea, peas, pinto beans, lentils, and other legumes. Lignans occur in flaxseeds (though flaxseed oil contains only small amounts).

Natural estrogen can be extracted from some foods, such as soy, and plant hormones from the wild yam have been extracted to create a progesterone-like cream. Some tests have shown that certain plant estrogens offer some relief from hot flashes of perimenopause and menopause, if the symptoms are mild. They are the subject of a great deal of ongoing research, as the medical community continues to test the safety and efficacy of these substances and to learn how their use compares with the effectiveness of traditional HRT in the treatment of symptoms of women with diminishing levels of hormone production.

Make sure to read some full-length texts that discuss these natural alternatives to HRT in complete detail. Use the information you gain in this chapter as a foundation for further research and discussions with your health care professional.

Soy and Isoflavones

Soy is a major source of a number of important vitamins and nutrients, and it is one of the primary sources for isoflavones—a type of plant estrogen. The North American Menopause Society has reported on a number of studies of the use of isoflavones and their role in managing menopausal health. (Some of the articles are listed in the References section of Appendix B.) Though some of the studies have been inconclusive and work continues in this area, many health and nutrition experts believe that soy has major benefits for treating some symptoms of menopause:

- The isoflavones in soy may help reduce LDL cholesterol and triglycerides while increasing HDL cholesterol levels.
- Many women find that soy reduces the occurrences and the severity of hot flashes.
- One study, conducted by Dr. Michael Scheiber and associates, reported in 2001, found that women who included whole soy foods in their diet had reductions in some of the key indicators for the onset of osteoporosis. (You can read this study online at *www.menopause.org* under abstract 85384 or see Appendix B for its print source in the NAMS journal.)
- Some women report that an increased intake of soy isoflavones helps alleviate their symptoms of vaginal dryness, though no long-term study has confirmed this.

Keep in mind that the type of soy you consume has a huge impact on the amount of symptom relief you may be able to expect. For example, raw, green soybeans contain the most isoflavones—as much as 150 milligrams per 100 grams of food—whereas soy hot dogs or breakfast sausage may contain only 3 or 4 milligrams. Most medical experts recommend that if you're using soy to manage menopause symptoms that you consume at least 100 milligrams per day (for 25 to 50 milligrams of isoflavones). In the Scheiber NAMS Fellowship study mentioned earlier, the participants ate whole soy foods containing 60 mg/d every day.

FACTS

Asian women, who eat a diet rich in soy products, have exceptionally low rates of hip and spine fractures and endometrial, breast, and ovarian cancers. Though the Asian diet is also low in red meat and saturated animal fats, researchers are working to track down possible connections between the consumption of soy isoflavones and the low rate of hormone-related conditions.

Soy products aren't calorie-free, but they tend to be low in fat, high in dietary fiber, and full of a range of important vitamins and minerals. Soy milk, tofu, tempeh, and imitation meat products such as burgers, sausage, and "unchicken" cutlets are just some of the readily available sources of soy. Soy sprouts, soy flour, and roasted soy beans also are rich sources of soy isoflavones.

Red clover is the second richest source of isoflavones. Though some herbal teas and compounds include red clover, it's more commonly taken as a plant extract. For more information about these ingredients, see Chapter 13, "Eating for a Healthy Menopause."

Black Cohosh

Black cohosh is perhaps one of the most popular herbal remedies used for the management of menopausal symptoms. Native American women have used its roots for centuries for relief of a number of symptoms associated with menstruation and menopause. The specific means by which it works is still the subject of intense study. German women have used black cohosh for decades as a means of diminishing hot flashes, depression, and other symptoms of menopause. In some studies, black cohosh was found to lower luteinizing hormone (LH) levels by binding to certain estrogen receptors. Double-blind tests conducted on Remifem, an over-the-counter supplement that contains black cohosh, found that some participants felt some relief from symptoms including hot flashes, depression-like symptoms, and occasional sleeplessness.

More studies are needed to determine if black cohosh is safe for women with breast cancer and other estrogen-sensitive cancers. Side effects of black cohosh include nausea, vomiting, dizziness, and at least one reported case of nocturnal seizures. Black cohosh should not be used during pregnancy, as it may cause miscarriage or premature birth. In menopause or perimenopause, its use is not recommended for more than six months.

Kava (sometimes called kava kava) has been used for some time to alleviate anxiety and tension, but it must be used with caution. Originally a plant of the Pacific islands, some natives used kava as an intoxicant. Its use has been linked to yellowing skin and mild stomach upset. Kava is addictive and can cause extreme drowsiness if you use it while drinking alcohol or taking antihistamines.

Gingko Biloba

Many women turn to gingko biloba supplements, extracted from the leaf of the gingko biloba tree, as treatment for the mental fogginess that seems to descend upon them as menopause approaches. Gingko biloba has been studied in placebo-controlled tests and shown to work better than a placebo at aiding memory and concentration. The National Institute on Aging has even studied the use of this extract in the treatment of Alzheimer's disease, though the results of those studies are not yet reported. However, gingko has been shown to improve circulation and may, therefore, aid the supply of nourishment to the brain through the circulatory system. Typical dosages of gingko are 40 to 80 milligrams (taken in capsule form) three times daily. Most sources indicate that you need to take this dosage for up to twelve weeks in order to feel the effect. Talk to your health care provider for information about dosage and appropriateness for your symptoms.

Finding Out about Other Herbs and Supplements

This chapter has listed only a few herbal compounds and nutritional supplements available for the treatment of menopausal symptoms. Others include:

- Chasteberry (Latin name, vitus agnus castus) is said to relieve hot flashes and vaginal dryness.
- Dong quai, believed by some to treat hot flashes, was found ineffective in recent studies and may increase the flow of menstrual blood. Other side effects include photosensitivity and photodermatitis (sun rash), and it may cause cancer or mutations or increase the effects of the drug warfarin (Coumadin—a frequently prescribed blood thinner) and antiplatelet agents.
- SAMe (S-Adenosylmethionine) is said to repair damaged cartilage for better joint health.
- Ginseng root is considered by many to aid menopausal symptoms, and may have a beneficial impact on mood through its mild stimulant effect.

You'll find many other examples of herbal compounds and nutritional supplements on most grocery and pharmacy shelves. As recommended earlier, do your own extensive research into any supplement before you begin using it. The Resources section of Appendix B offers a variety of print and online sources for more information. And, as always, talk to your health care provider for a full understanding of how these products may work for the treatment of your symptoms.

SSENTIALS Many women claim to have found real relief from hot flashes, anxiety, and other menopausal symptoms through acupressure and therapeutic massage. In acupressure, a therapist places pressure on the body at the same meridian points used in acupuncture. Many types of therapeutic massage operate on the principle that stimulating the body's circulation and lymph gland production boosts health.

Therapeutic Programs

Women in the United States are learning that many of the medical traditions from other cultures have some use for the management of menopausal symptoms. And some traditional Western therapies such as counseling and cognitive therapy are incredibly effective for treating some of the most debilitating symptoms of menopause, including mood swings, irritability, and depression. Some of the therapeutic programs women have found useful in treating symptoms of perimenopause and menopause are:

- Acupuncture is an ancient Chinese therapy that involves rotating fine needles until they enter the skin at specific points on the body. In a 1995 test reported by the North American Menopause Society in the journal *Menopause*, women treated with both electrically aided and traditional acupuncture showed a significant decrease in hot flashes, lasting up to three months after treatment. The National Institute of Health Consensus Development Panel on Acupuncture issued a statement saying that acupuncture may be helpful in managing conditions such as headache, fibromyalgia, osteoarthritis, and cramps—conditions some women face in perimenopause and menopause. This alternative treatment option is still being studied for its applications in the management of menopause symptoms.
- Breathing regulation, where women are trained to breathe deeply and slowly (sometimes called paced respiration), has also shown some promise in reducing hot flashes and aiding relaxation. For perimenopausal and menopausal women suffering from hot flashes, anxiety, and panic attacks, this technique can be particularly useful. Perhaps due to the same calm, slow respiratory technique taught in practices such as yoga and meditation, some women report those practices have also helped them in alleviating anxiety as well as the frequency and intensity of hot flashes.
- Biofeedback is a technique in which individuals are trained to monitor breathing, heart rate, and blood pressure, and then change those functions through relaxation techniques or visual imagery. Studies on biofeedback have been ongoing since the 1970s, and some have

indicated that biofeedback techniques can help women control hot flashes and stress incontinence.

- Cognitive therapy—a type of talk therapy—has long been used to help individuals overcome depression; many women find it an invaluable tool for coming to terms with the changing realities of their lives and health as they approach and enter menopause. Cognitive therapy focuses on helping the individual learn to see the connection between a pattern of negative thought and depression. As you learn to replace negative thoughts with positive ones, you can break damaging thinking patterns that contribute to deepening, ongoing depression and anxiety. Many women become the victims of constant negative thinking as they approach menopause; cognitive therapy can help break that pattern and thereby alleviate the moodiness, lethargy, irritability, sadness, and insomnia that it can cause.

Lifestyle Changes for a Healthier Menopause

This chapter has saved the most important alternative for combating menopausal symptoms for last. Lifestyle choices, including eliminating certain substances from your life; exercising regularly; eating a healthy, well-balanced diet with appropriate vitamin and mineral supplements; managing weight; and getting regular aerobic and weight-bearing exercise are essential for any woman entering menopause, whether or not she chooses to use HRT or alternative treatments to manage symptoms. Throughout this chapter you've been advised to seek the advice of a trusted health care professional (or two, or three). When you sit down with that individual, the following are some of the first questions he or she will ask:

- "How's your diet? Do you take any vitamins?"
- "Do you get any regular form of exercise? What kind? How often?"
- "Do you smoke? Do you use any nonprescription drugs or stimulants? How much alcohol do you consume?"
- "How much stress are you under?"

So—use the following five-point plan to minimize the number and severity of your perimenopausal and menopausal symptoms, maintain optimal health through menopause, and set the stage for your healthy, active, enjoyable postmenopausal life:

FACTS

Concentrate on what you can eat now, and experiment with foods you may not have tried before. Baked parsnips and sweet potatoes, for example, are flavorful, rich dishes that offer good sources of fiber, vitamins, and minerals. And these foods are naturally sweet, so you can throw out the miniature marshmallows.

1. **Eat a heart-healthy, well-balanced diet with the vitamin, mineral, and nutrient balance recommended for a woman at your stage of life.** Feeding your body properly is the most important thing you can do to manage your menopause—and your health. Limit your salt, animal fat, and simple carbohydrate intake. Eat plenty of green leafy vegetables, root vegetables, and fresh and dried fruit. Make sure your diet includes ample quantities of vitamin C, vitamin D, vitamin E, and calcium. Now is the time to start reading labels and eating as though your life depends on it. (See Chapter 13.)

2. **Get regular physical activity that includes both weight-bearing and aerobic exercise.** Thirty minutes a day, four or more days a week, of walking, bike riding, swimming, or other exercise can keep your heart and lungs healthy, your mind alert, and your spirits up. (See Chapter 14.)

3. **Manage your weight.** Obesity has become a national epidemic. According to the National Institute of Diabetes and Digestive and Kidney Diseases, more than 50 percent of all Americans are overweight. And even if you've never suffered from weight problems in the past, your body could begin to put on pounds in perimenopause. As you approach middle age, your metabolism slows down, so you burn fewer calories—even at rest. If you work in a sedentary job and if your idea of a good time involves a recliner, a remote control, and a bowl of cheese doodles, you might be feeding

one of the most dangerous symptoms of menopause—weight gain. You need to gear up for battle and commit to doing all you can to maintain a healthy weight; talk to your doctor or health care professional for advice on the program that might work best for you.

4. **Stop smoking and don't overindulge in alcohol.** If you smoke, you need to stop now—for your health and for the health of anyone who lives with you. Death by lung cancer, heart disease, or emphysema isn't pretty, quick, or painless, so why increase your risks of contracting those diseases? If you need help quitting (and most people do), talk to your health care provider or contact the American Lung Association (ALA) at ✆(800) LUNG-USA. If you have Internet access, you can use the ALA's smoking cessation program at *www.lungusa.org*. And manage your use of alcohol, too. Most medical experts now agree that moderate drinking—one or two drinks a day—can be healthy (if you aren't taking medications or fighting conditions that prohibit alcohol consumption). If you drink more than a few alcoholic drinks every day, you may be contributing to your high blood pressure. Alcohol isn't exactly calorie-free either—calories add up, whether you chew them or not. Moderation is the key.

5. **Manage your stress.** Stress is damaging to your health in so many ways; it can cause everything from upset stomach to depression to heart disease. And if it did nothing to harm your health (which it always does), stress dramatically diminishes the quality of your life. Now is the time to learn to enjoy the days and people that make up your life. Avoid the stressors you can avoid, diminish those you can't avoid, and add relaxation and rest to offset the damage of dealing with stress. Exercise, diet, ample rest, and following a regular relaxation technique are your best stress busters. (See Chapter 18.)

Keeping Your Eyes on the Prize

As you approach menopause, you may find that you gain a greater appreciation every day of your health and its precious gifts. No one can stop the aging process—and who would want to? But as our bodies change, as the medical profession uncovers new treatment strategies, as science continually works to forge new understandings of our body and its processes, everything we know about menopause evolves. As you evaluate and follow treatment options for maintaining your physical and emotional health throughout this time in your life, remember to keep an open mind and remain curious.

Remember that your goal with any menopause management plan is to maintain your physical and emotional health and to alleviate symptoms that threaten either. Don't grow complacent; the strategy you choose today may need rethinking a year down the road.

Follow medical developments, closely monitor your symptoms and treatment reactions, and continue to work with your health care provider to make sure that the plan you've chosen is the best option for you today. Nothing stays the same, and you can't afford to assume that today's treatment decision will still be the best choice throughout all of your tomorrows.

CHAPTER 13

Eating for a Healthy Menopause

A healthy diet, supplemented with recommended vitamins and minerals, is your best tool for controlling or preventing some of the most damaging and debilitating conditions that affect women during and after menopause.

Your Nutritional Needs after Age Forty

A woman's body goes through significant changes as it approaches menopause; estrogen production slows dramatically, muscle mass decreases as fat deposits increase, metabolism slows down, body tissues—including those of the heart and circulatory system—lose elasticity, and the body begins reabsorbing bone cells at a faster rate than it produces them. For many women, stiff, aching joints; mood swings; feelings of lethargy; and insomnia join the list of physiological symptoms that accompany perimenopause. All of these symptoms contribute to serious health risks stemming from two oddly disparate yet closely linked conditions—overweight and undernourishment.

The health risks of perimenopause and menopause include an increased risk of cardiovascular disease, diabetes, and osteoporosis. Add to these risks the serious health problems associated with overweight and obesity, and the challenges of maintaining your health as you approach menopause become painfully clear. Meeting these challenges requires a diet designed to both manage weight and boost nutrition.

FACTS

Does it seem as if you're eating the same amount of food you've always eaten, yet you're gaining weight? Your perception may be true; as women age, their metabolism slows down and they burn fewer calories in everything they do. So, if your body is burning less energy while consuming the same amount of fuel, you will gain weight.

Many people go through life using their diets for everything but nutrition. They try one fad diet after another to lose weight; they load up on junk food and high-fat ice cream and chocolate as "food therapy" for overcoming anger, sadness, and disappointment; they choose foods based on convenience, portability, and easy cleanup. Though you may get by eating a shabby diet for a while, some time around your early forties, you might begin to feel the negative impact of bad eating habits. And even if you've always maintained a relatively healthy diet, you still may not be giving your changing body the nutrition it needs now.

What are the nutritional needs of women during and after menopause? Nutrition experts from the Institute of Medicine recommend these daily amounts of vitamins and minerals:

NUTRIENT (UNIT)	DAILY AMOUNT
Calcium (mg)	1,500 (1,200 with HRT)
Magnesium (mg/d)	320
Iron (mg/d)	5
Zinc (mg/d)	8
Iodine (µg/d)	150
Selenium (µg/d)	55
Vitamin A (µg/d)	700
Vitamin E (mg/d)	15
Vitamin D (µg/d)	10
Vitamin K (µg/d)	90
Vitamin C (mg/d)	75
Riboflavin (mg/d)	1.1
Thiamin (mg/d)	1.1
Niacin (mg/d)	14
Vitamin B_6 (mg/d)	1.5
Folate (mg/d)	400
Vitamin B_{12} (µg/d)	2.4

(Table taken from the American College of Obstetricians and Gynecologists patient education publication AP151, *A Healthy Diet*)

Nutritional Boosts for Women over Forty

Women approaching menopause have to pay special attention to the types and quantities of nutrients they consume each day. The following list includes just some of the special nutritional concerns for women at the age of menopause (remember that these amounts are general recommendations; women taking certain medications or combating specific conditions may need to take more or less, depending upon their doctor or health care professional's recommendations).

FACTS

Free-radical damage to LDL cholesterol causes it to adhere to the walls of your arteries. The antioxidant effect of vitamin E stops the action of these free radicals, and therefore helps prevent the onset of heart disease.

- **Calcium is a woman's best friend as she approaches the age of menopause.** Because the risk of developing osteoporosis increases as estrogen levels decrease, women need to be particularly careful to consume the recommended amount of calcium every day. If you're postmenopausal and taking HRT, you should consume 1,200 mg daily; if you're not taking HRT, and for all women sixty-five years of age or over, 1,500 mg is a must. Calcium is in milk, yogurt, cheese, and other dairy products, as well as in fortified fruit juices. (See Eating for Strong Bones in Chapter 8.) Nevertheless, you may need to use supplements to get the full recommended amount.
- **Vitamin D is an essential partner to the calcium in your diet.** Vitamin D helps your body absorb and use calcium, and you can get 100 of the 400 IU recommended daily amount in one eight-ounce glass of skim milk. Some juices and certain brands of calcium supplements are also available with added vitamin D.
- **Fiber is an important part of every woman's diet, and it's particularly important for women reaching the age of menopause.** Women should eat 25 to 30 grams of fiber daily. Soluble fiber, found in fruit, vegetables, dried beans, barley, and oats, helps keep cholesterol levels low and can help prevent heart disease and lower the risk of stroke. Insoluble fiber, the type found in complex carbohydrates such as whole grains and the skins of fruits and vegetables, provides bulk that helps keep your digestive system on track and can help prevent colon cancer.
- **Antioxidants, including vitamins A, C, E, and beta carotene, are vitamins found in a number of brightly colored fruits and vegetables.** These are now considered important tools in warding off heart disease and some cancers, and may even reduce the deterioration of macular degeneration (age-related vision loss). Antioxidants work to stop the effects of oxidation within your body by protecting your body tissue

from the effect of free radicals—molecules in your body that lack an electron, and therefore "steal" one from other body cells. Like rustproofing treatments for your car, antioxidants block these free radicals from damaging your body's tissues. Squash, sweet potatoes, spinach, mangos, tomatoes, red peppers, oranges, blueberries, and peaches are just some of the fresh fruit and vegetable sources of antioxidants. Chocolate may also provide some antioxidant benefits, but don't forget about calories when adding it to your diet.

- **Soy and other phytoestrogens can have a beneficial effect on your body as its natural hormone production slows down.** Even though phytoestrogens are dramatically less potent than the body's natural estrogens, they can help alleviate some hormonal symptoms, such as hot flashes. Soy protein has real benefits for your heart; eating 25 mg daily can help lower LDL cholesterol by 5 to 10 percent. You find soy protein in soy milk (7 grams in 1 cup), veggie burger mix (11 grams in ½ cup), tofu (10 grams in 4 ounces), and roasted soy nuts (17 grams in ¼ cup), among other foods.

- **Omega-3 fatty acids are found in fish, nuts, flaxseed, tofu, and soybean and canola oils.** These essential fatty acids help nourish the hair, nails, and skin, but that isn't their only role in preserving health during menopause. New studies have shown that omega-3 fatty acids offer a number of benefits for cardiovascular health. The American Heart Association (AHA) reports that increasing the consumption of omega-3 fatty acids can benefit people who have pre-existing cardiovascular disease as well as those with healthy hearts and circulatory systems— especially when those fatty acids are consumed as part of a balanced diet. The AHA recommends two three-ounce servings of salmon, tuna, mackerel, herring, or other fatty fish every week.

FACTS

According to the AHA, older Americans are less likely to die from cardiovascular disease if they eat at least one serving (3 ounces cooked weight) of fatty fish every week. Many deaths due to heart disease are the result of arrhythmias, and omega-3 fatty acids may help reduce their occurrence. One study showed a 44 percent reduction in death due to heart attack among fatty fish-eating participants.

Get It from Your Plate, Not a Pill

The best nutrition comes from food—not supplements. Though even a well-balanced diet might require the added benefit of vitamin and mineral supplements, those supplements should be used only to "top off" the nutrients supplied by food. If you aren't sure whether or not your current diet is giving you all of the nutrients you need, your doctor or health care professional can test your vitamin and mineral levels. Then, he or she can help you decide what (if any) supplements you need. A multivitamin mineral supplement is recommended, however, for anyone who is dieting, under stress, recovering from a recent illness, suffering from a chronic condition, or trying to boost his or her immune system.

Don't forget the importance of drinking at least two to three quarts of water every day. Water is essential for cooling your body, transmitting nutrients throughout your system, and hydrating all of your body's tissues. When you're dieting and/or exercising, you must be especially careful to drink ample amounts of water throughout the day.

Eating for Weight Management

Some changes that accompany age are linked to hormonal loss, while others appear to be linked to other natural processes of aging. Though medical science continues to study the causes and effects of the changes women experience in middle age, some facts remain clear and indisputable:

- As women age, they tend to lose muscle tissue and gain fat tissue.
- As women age, their metabolism slows down.
- As women age, their body fat is redistributed to their abdomen and midsection, unless they take estrogen replacement therapy, which helps maintain the traditional female fat distribution; in other words, keeping you looking pear shaped instead of apple shaped.

These facts aren't a signal that women are doomed to become fat and dumpy in middle age. However, as you consider how to construct a healthy diet for your midlife transition, you need to keep these realities in mind.

The Facts about Midlife Weight Gain

As your metabolism slows, you burn fewer calories; as your percentage of muscle tissue decreases and fat tissue increases, your body consumes fewer calories. These facts together mean that, all other things remaining equal, if you continue to consume the same number of calories through perimenopause and menopause that you consumed when you were premenopausal, you can expect to gain weight.

In one study conducted by the University of Pittsburgh, women gained an average of 2 kilograms (about 4.4 pounds) over three years of their menopausal transition. By eight years after menopause, the women gained an average of 5.5 kilograms (a little over 12 pounds). Though all women won't gain this much weight during menopause, many will—and some will gain even more. Without question, exercise is a must for controlling midlife weight gain. (See Chapter 14.) But eating a healthy, well-balanced diet is your other weapon to fight off this potentially deadly problem.

FACTS

To calculate how many calories you burn every day, multiply your weight by fifteen (if you're moderately active) or thirteen (if you get little exercise). The answer represents the approximate number of calories you burn during an average day.

Don't misunderstand the message here; a slight weight gain at midlife isn't necessarily a health risk. Women's bodies change during their transition, and the addition of one or two pounds is an expected part of that change. But overweight and obesity—as determined by a Body Mass Index (BMI) of 25 or higher—are conditions associated with all sorts of health risks for men and women alike, including high cholesterol and high blood pressure. The heavier you are, the harder you must work to move, and the less you feel like exercising. Being overweight can make you feel lethargic, depressed, and powerless—feelings no woman needs during her transition through menopause. There is some truth to the ironic observation: "The more you exercise, the more you feel like exercising; the less you exercise, the less you feel like exercising."

And the redistribution of body fat to your abdomen and midsection has dangerous implications. A large amount of abdominal fat is considered a high-risk factor for the development of diabetes and coronary heart disease.

ESSENTIALS

Though slowing hormone production contributes to all of these (and many other) facts of life for most women over the age of forty, just beginning an HRT regimen without making any other adjustments is not going to solve all your problems. Make lifestyle changes—a healthy diet and ample exercise—part of any health management plan.

Temporary or Fad Diet Plans Aren't the Answer

Remember, when you read the word "diet" in this book, don't think about "the incredible all banana and cabbage weight-loss miracle" you read about on the Internet. Adopting and maintaining a healthy diet does not mean starving yourself or combining certain foods to magically block fat from being absorbed into your system. Long-term weight loss requires that you change your eating habits for good—not just until you drop that extra five or ten pounds. A healthy diet for long-term weight loss involves common sense: lowering your fat intake, lowering your simple sugar intake, and decreasing your portion size. In general, you must eliminate 3,500 calories from your system in order to lose a single pound of body fat. By lowering your calorie intake and increasing the number of calories you burn through a regular exercise program, you will lose weight. Stick to this program as a lifestyle change, and you will maintain a healthy weight.

When you find yourself turning to food for the wrong reasons—to alleviate loneliness, boredom, fatigue, and so on—stop and think of something that will really help. Call a friend, take a short walk around the block, pick up a book, go to a movie, work on a crossword puzzle, work in the garden, or write in a journal. Food won't solve any problem other than physical (not emotional or spiritual) hunger.

Good Eating Habits Aid Weight Control

A key component of managing weight gain during menopause is to develop good eating habits. Again, it really doesn't matter what's always worked for you before; your body is changing, and your eating patterns have to change, too, if you want to avoid excess weight gain. The following suggestions may help you:

- **Avoid fast food.** No matter how easy it is to grab a meal from the drive-through window or have it hustled to your door by a delivery person, fast food is packed with all of the things you don't need to eat, such as saturated fats, sugar, cholesterol, and salt. For the whopping 1,000 calories you may consume with that double bacon cheeseburger, you're getting precious little nourishment. Plan menus, shop for fresh produce, and learn to pack your lunch (with daytime snacks). If you have time on the weekend to prepare and bag fruit and vegetable salads, you can enjoy them through the week.

- **Try to enjoy your meals.** Sit down at a table whenever possible, and put your food on a plate rather than eating it out of your hand. Do not eat standing over the kitchen sink, and do not walk down the street eating a breakfast burrito. Take your time; look at the food you're eating, smell it, and pay attention to each bite. Then, you're more likely to know when you're full. Shoveling food down while you stare at the television, drive to work, or read the paper by the kitchen sink is a sure ticket to overeating. If you really love to eat, do it with purpose.

- **Don't wait until you're starving to eat.** Try to eat small meals spaced out throughout the day. Eat a light breakfast, have a piece of fruit or a cup of yogurt midmorning, eat a healthy lunch, have a midafternoon snack, then enjoy a light dinner. The hungrier you are when you eat, the more likely you are to wolf down more food than you need. And the less cause you give your fat cells to get ready to sock it away. However, if you aren't hungry, don't eat. One of the biggest diet myths is that one absolutely has to have at least three meals a day. If you are not normally hungry in the morning, do not force yourself to eat breakfast.

- **Avoid eating late at night or right before going to bed.** Many people in the United States eat very little during the day, then pack it away from the time they reach home until they go to bed at night—a very bad eating habit. You're active and at work during the day, so that's when you need your fuel. By the time you go to bed, your body should be ready to rest—not attempting to digest several pounds of recently consumed food.

- **Don't try to become a "food reformist" overnight.** If you need a dramatic diet makeover, take it in small steps. Give up one or two of your worst food habits at a time, and introduce healthy substitutes slowly. Start small—buy thin-sliced whole-wheat bread instead of white, try a new squash recipe, declare a weekly salad night, or skip the cookies and have a handful of grapes. If you don't want to completely turn your back on your favorite junk food, try limiting your quantities— maybe even set up a timeline, with a planned withdrawal period. Don't punish yourself about your eating habits—just work to make them better.

- **Keep a food journal for two weeks, where you write down everything you eat—including quantities!** It's essential that you know approximately how much you're eating. Many people think, "Oh, well, I had a spoonful of mashed potatoes, but that doesn't count." The fact is that everything you eat counts and your spoonful might be one-half cup, a cup, or more. That crisp green salad takes on some hefty calories when you ladle on the dressing; get out the tablespoon and measure how much you use (and check the label for calorie count). Weigh it, measure it, write it down. Then, you have a better idea of the amount of diet reformation you need.

- **Pay attention to portion sizes.** A protein serving should weigh about three ounces and be about the same size as a pack of cards. A serving of pasta is around one-half cup, not the plateful they bring you in most restaurants. One slice of bread or one cup of flaked cereal is one serving. A serving of fruit is one medium-sized fruit or one-half cup of fruit juice; vegetable serving sizes are one-half to one cup of raw or cooked vegetables.

If you aren't accustomed to eating raw fruit and vegetables, add them gradually to your diet. These foods are essential to maintaining good health, but your system has to have time to adjust to digesting them. If you suddenly load your system up with an unusually high level of raw fruit and vegetables, you can have stomach pains, gas, and other gastrointestinal complaints.

Sane, Simple Guidelines for Healthy Eating

Putting together a healthy diet doesn't require that you have a Ph.D. in nutrition, a live-in cook, or a personal shopper. It just requires a little bit of education and a commitment to spend a little more time buying and preparing the right foods. This book isn't going to outline a week's worth of healthy meals; plenty of books do that already, and anyway, the choices are much too varied to be presented here. But here's what your food choices should represent, every single day:

- Six or more servings of whole grains
- Five or six servings of a variety of fresh fruit and vegetables
- Two or three servings of protein foods such as fish, lean animal foods, beans, nuts, and seeds

With those very general guidelines, incorporate these dos and don'ts:

- **Limit your intake of fats; total fat intake should be under 30 percent of all of your calories.** Avoid transfats and saturated fats. Fats in nuts, fatty fish, olive oil, flaxseed oil, and canola oil are healthier for you than are those in animal fats, shortening, and hydrogenated vegetable oils.

- **Eat a wide variety of fruit and vegetables, of a variety of deep, rich colors.** Green leafy vegetables, oranges, tomatoes, squash and blueberries are some of the low-fat, high-antioxidant foods you should include in your diet. Most produce sections carry a wide variety of vegetables and fruit, so why stick with the same old stuff you grew up eating? Try new things, experiment, and focus on nutrition.

- **Limit your intake of salt; high sodium levels contribute to high blood pressure and too much salt actually inhibits the natural flavors of the food you eat.** If your usual routine includes salting your food before you taste it, work on breaking it. Taste your food before you add any salt. Also, consider a salt substitute, particularly if you are on a sodium-restricted diet.

- **Try to add "meno-healthy" foods into your diet.** Remember the benefits of fatty fishes—salmon, tuna, and so on—and eat some twice a week. Add soy to your diet, whether through soy milk, tofu, or roasted soy nut snacks. Don't dismiss these foods without trying them. They're high in nutrients and low in fat.

Often, menopausal women feel that they're being forced to give up the foods they love as some sort of punishment for their age and sex. Your diet is one of the things you have complete control over, so be proud of your decision to eat the foods that will keep your body strong and healthy.

- **Be sensible about caffeine and alcohol consumption.** Caffeine has been shown to leach calcium from the body, and it can aggravate conditions such as elevated blood pressure, anxiety, and tension. If you don't want to stop drinking caffeine altogether (your best choice), consider switching from coffee to green tea—many green teas have only small quantities of caffeine and are rich in antioxidants. Don't drink more than one or two alcoholic beverages a day. Excess alcohol leads to a number of health problems, and alcohol is loaded with calories. Though most health experts agree that wine has antioxidant qualities and can actually be good for you, keep your consumption of it low. You'll gain less weight and feel better.

Your Own Revolution

The food you eat plays a major role in determining your long-term health. As you approach midlife, you have an excellent opportunity to re-evaluate your food choices and adopt a diet that will help ensure a long, healthy, active life ahead. Food is a great joy and an important part of many of our favorite family rituals—you should enjoy eating. Maintaining a healthy diet doesn't require that you demonize every donut or treat each stack of pancakes as if it were a ticking time bomb. It simply means making thoughtful choices about the foods you eat, and using food as a means to accomplish your health goals.

You'll never have a reason to regret improving your nutrition. No matter how many miraculous new medicines and treatments medical science develops for correcting the effects of disease or minimizing the changes that occur as we age, nothing will ever replace the marvelous health benefits of a well-balanced diet and regular exercise.

CHAPTER 14

Building Exercise into Your Menopause Plan

By the time they reach the age of perimenopause, most women have developed some strong attitudes about exercise. Either they exercise regularly and can't imagine doing without it, or they've determined that exercise just isn't for them. Exercise combats many of the physical and emotional symptoms of perimenopause and menopause, and—in combination with a healthy, varied, well-balanced diet—it's your best alternative for aging slowly, gracefully, and healthfully.

Why You Need Exercise Now

A woman's body is primed for weight gain in midlife. Although becoming unfit is never a good idea, it can seem particularly damaging at this time in a woman's life. Near the age of menopause, metabolism slows down and muscle tissue diminishes, while fat deposits develop around the center of the body. Hormonal fluctuations can result in a variety of symptoms, including mood swings, feelings of lethargy, hot flashes, and heightened anxiety and depression. Caught in a vicious circle of diminishing fitness, some women find themselves wanting to eat more and exercise less, just when their bodies need the opposite prescription.

Even those women who maintain the same level of physical activity and food intake through menopause can expect to gain weight and lose muscle tone. This decline in fitness makes even a long-practiced exercise program less effective than it used to be and more difficult to adhere to. In the Healthy Women's Study conducted at the University of Pittsburgh, researchers found that by eight years after menopause, the women in their study gained an average of twelve pounds. The strongest predictor for that weight gain was decreased physical activity.

FACTS

According to the Surgeon General's Report on Physical Activity and Health, physical inactivity is more common among women than men. The report states that more than 60 percent of women in the United States get too little exercise, and 25 percent get no regular exercise at all.

Does all of this mean that you're destined for fatness, not fitness, as you approach menopause? Absolutely not! These realities of midlife change simply mean that whatever your current fitness practices may be, they probably need an overhaul when you enter perimenopause. If you've never followed an exercise program, if you've tried and abandoned regular exercise—even if you currently are following an exercise program that's been working for you over the past several years—you need a new fitness plan. Following are some reasons why you need exercise now.

- Your workday may be less physically demanding than at previous times in your life. At midlife, you may have become a "desk potato," as your job has advanced to include more managerial duties and fewer tasks that require legwork. Although you may feel as though you are constantly in motion, in reality you may only be going from sitting down to standing up more often, and not actually burning any calories.

- Your stress levels may be on the rise. As your career advances, the demands it places on you can increase accordingly. Economic and social upheavals, concerns over adolescent children and/or aging parents, and the onset of your own age-related aches and pains are just some of the stress makers you may face at midlife. Aside from its psychological toll, stress can cause chronic pain in your muscles, feed insomnia and fatigue, and trigger weight gain.

As you pass age forty, your risk of developing a number of life-threatening age-related diseases begins to rise. Heart disease, diabetes, high blood pressure, elevated cholesterol levels, osteoporosis, and certain cancers are some of the deadly conditions that menopausal women must guard against. Physical inactivity is a prime indicator for many of them.

- After age fifty, your joint health and physical motor abilities can begin to deteriorate. As you lose balance and coordination, you become more likely to fall—and less likely to participate in physical activities. Knees and hips can become stiff and painful, further damaging your interest or ability in leading a healthy, active life. The less active you are, the faster (and further) these conditions develop. If your eyesight is worsening as well, sports such as tennis and golf may become less pleasurable.

- Your body shape and your body image may be changing at menopause. As your body takes on the natural contours of middle age, you may feel that you no longer have any control of your body's condition. A lot of people say that they just feel like giving up, but throwing in the towel on fitness now can set the stage for a continuous decline in health, physical capability, and emotional well-being.

Exercise Can Save Your Life

A number of life-threatening diseases become greater health risks for women as they approach the age of menopause. Here are just some of the potentially life-saving benefits of following a regular, sustained program of exercise:

Never begin any kind of exercise program without first discussing the details with your doctor or health care provider. Your health care professional can help assess your capacity for exercise and what type of exercise program might be the most beneficial for your particular needs.

- **Exercise makes your heart healthier:** Your heart is a muscle that grows weak with continued inactivity. The walls of an inactive woman's heart grow thin and are less effective at pumping blood throughout her system. Regular, aerobic exercise builds the heart along with other muscle tissues in the body. The walls of a physically active woman's heart grow thicker and stronger; her heart is healthier and does a better job of pumping nourishing blood throughout her circulatory system, especially under periods of physical or emotional stress.
- **Exercise helps keep cholesterol levels down and arterial flow up:** Even moderate levels of regular exercise can lower the level of LDL cholesterol in a woman's bloodstream. LDL cholesterol is responsible for the fatty deposits that collect on the walls of arteries, contributing to high blood pressure, heart attack, and stroke. A regular program of aerobic exercise contributes to clean, clear arteries that allow ample supplies of fresh, oxygenated blood to feed the heart and other body tissues.
- **Exercise helps prevent diabetes:** Diabetes is on the rise in America. The CDC estimates that diabetes among Americans increased by 49 percent between 1990 and 2000. Obesity and inactivity are recognized as the primary culprits in the proliferation of the disease. Numerous studies show that physical activity in combination with a healthy diet

can prevent or delay the onset of type 2 diabetes, even in people who are at high risk for contracting the disease.

- **Exercise builds strong bones:** Women who participate in little or no regular physical activity can lose at least 1 percent of their bone mass each year—even before menopause. Participating in regular weight-bearing exercise, including walking, can slow and even reverse this bone loss.

- **Exercise can help prevent some types of cancer:** The American Cancer Society reports that new research has shown that even moderate physical activity can lower breast cancer risk. And, because obesity is considered a risk factor for developing endometrial cancer, exercise helps reduce the risk for that disease. Regular physical activity also reduces risks for developing colon cancer, a growing threat for women age fifty and over.

- **Exercise may help prevent or slow the development of Alzheimer's disease:** A 1998 study conducted by researchers at Case Western Reserve University School of Medicine and University Hospitals of Cleveland found that people who exercise regularly are less likely to develop Alzheimer's disease. Physically active people who do develop the disease are more likely to develop it late in life and experience a slower progression of symptoms.

- **Exercise improves mental well-being in general:** Moderate exercise causes the brain to release more endorphins—naturally occurring substances that resemble opiates, and are considered to be the neurotransmitters that make you feel good and happy. The sense of satisfaction that you get from completing an exercise routine will carry over into the rest of your day, and may help with the discipline you need to stick to your healthful diet.

FACTS

Over 250,000 people suffer from hip fractures every year in the United States. Porous bones, lack of muscle strength, ailing knee joints, and reduced balance and coordination all contribute to these injuries— conditions related to physical inactivity. If you think you're too young to start worrying about these problems, think again. Many women begin suffering from walking impairments as early as age fifty.

Managing Symptoms of Menopause

A healthy heart, strong bones, and a better chance for freedom from cancer, diabetes, heart disease, and other debilitating and fatal illnesses are all pretty persuasive reasons to start exercising at any time of life. But menopausal women have still more to gain from following a program of regular, sustained exercise. Physical activity has been shown to help tame many of the menopausal symptoms that women hate most, including insomnia, fatigue, anxiety, and mood swings. Regular, moderate exercise has been shown to reduce stress, help alleviate the severity of panic disorders, and elevate feelings of well-being. Here's a closer look at some of the menopause symptom-management benefits of exercise:

- **Exercise boosts your metabolism:** As you exercise, your metabolism speeds up, and it remains elevated for a while even after you stop exercising. The more energetic and sustained your exercise, the longer the metabolic boost lasts. An elevated metabolism helps your body burn more calories, which can help you lose weight.

- **Exercise may improve cognitive function:** In research conducted at Duke University and reported in the January 2001 issue of *The Journal of Aging and Physical Activity* regular exercise was shown to improve significantly the cognitive functions of individuals over the age of fifty. In the study, participants who completed thirty minutes of aerobic exercise (walking, jogging, bicycling) three times a week experienced significant improvements in cognitive functions such as memory, planning, organization, and intellectual multitasking. Though researchers haven't determined exactly how exercise works to improve brain functions, they believe the improvements may be attributed to increased blood and oxygen flow to the brain.

- **Exercise relieves depression:** In the same Duke University study that revealed the brain-boosting benefits of regular exercise, researchers also found that the relatively modest exercise program gave participants significant relief from the symptoms of major depression. In fact, the original goal of the study, called SMILE (Standard Medical Intervention and Long-term Exercise), was to determine how regular physical activity compared to antidepressant drug therapy in treating individuals diagnosed with major depressive disorder. After sixteen weeks, researchers found that those participants who practiced the regular exercise program had the same level of symptom relief as did those taking the antidepressant drugs. Exercise is known to trigger the body's production of endorphins—chemicals that can boost mood and alleviate tension—but researchers are still trying to determine all of the ways exercise works to ease depression.

FACTS

Body fat around the throat can contribute to snoring, a condition that exacts a toll on both the snorer and those who hear her snoring at night. Exercise can help reduce body fat, and thereby help eliminate or reduce the severity of snoring and the more serious condition of sleep apnea—a disorder in which the sleeper experiences interruptions in air intake that result in snoring and periodic breathing cessation.

- **Exercise helps you sleep:** Many women entering menopause are plagued by insomnia, and countless studies have shown that participating in a regular exercise program can help women go to sleep more quickly and experience fewer sleep interruptions. (Don't exercise right before going to bed, however; exercise leaves you feeling pumped up and can make it difficult to fall asleep right away.)
- **Exercise may help prevent hot flashes:** Though no study to date has shown that exercise can stop hot flashes, many studies have shown that hot flashes and other vasomotor symptoms are less common in physically active postmenopausal women than in those who get little or no physical exercise.
- **Exercise improves your endurance and makes you feel like moving:** Women approaching menopause can experience muscle loss and joint pain that effectively discourages them from doing the things they enjoy in life—gardening, dancing, even walking. Regular exercise strengthens muscles, builds endurance, and improves joint mobility and stability, enabling women to remain active and engaged in life.

Your Unique Fitness Goals

Maintaining your fitness is the most important component of your menopause management plan. Whether you intend to use HRT or an alternative therapy, whether you have special risk factors for specific diseases or no personal or genetic-based risks, whether you experience all or none of the physical and emotional symptoms of perimenopause and menopause, fitness maintenance is your overriding priority now and for the remaining years of your life. If you remain strong, active, and well-nourished, you will experience fewer symptoms. You'll have greater resistance to any illness or disease, and you'll progress faster and more successfully through treatments for any condition that does develop.

FACTS

Your genes matter. In a report published by the President's Council on Fitness, researchers found that genetic heritability for body fatness is 25 percent or more, muscle fitness 20 to 40 percent, and 10 to 25 percent for cardiovascular fitness. The study also found that some individuals benefit as much as ten times more than others from the same levels of physical activity.

But what does fitness mean? This question has important implications for you as you and your health provider form an exercise and diet plan designed to achieve that all-important goal of health fitness. There is no single universally accepted definition for the term "fitness," because of the vast differences in individuals' genetic makeup. People inherit certain physical characteristics that affect body composition, cardiovascular actions, and other important measures of good health. Heredity also plays a role in how individuals respond to exercise. But your heavy parents or grandparents have not doomed you to being physically out of shape or unresponsive to exercise. The exercise program that's right for your next-door neighbor, or even your sister, may not be right for you. Your individual hereditary and lifestyle factors determine how your body looks and responds at its peak fitness condition.

Your doctor or health care professional can help you determine what fitness goals best fit you as an individual. Most health professionals assess fitness based on the following six factors:

- Cardiorespiratory performance or aerobic endurance
- Muscular strength and endurance
- Flexibility
- Body composition—the amount of body fat and its distribution
- Bone density and strength
- Metabolic balance (how the body metabolizes glucose and insulin, blood lipid levels, and other metabolic actions)

Because individual genetic makeup plays a major role in body fat composition and distribution, medical authorities carefully assess individuals when determining realistic goals for fat reduction. In addition to calculating BMI, your health care professional may perform a skin fold test to determine your body fat levels.

Your health care professional can help you not only determine healthy goals for your weight, body measurement, endurance, and cardiovascular performance, but also monitor your progress and suggest periodic revisions in your exercise program to keep it working for you.

What Kind of Exercise Do You Need?

As unique as your individual fitness markers may be, any complete exercise program includes components aimed at improving three basic types of fitness: aerobic fitness, strength, and flexibility. The following sections take a closer look at each of these types of fitness and some examples of specific exercises that contribute to their development.

Aerobic Fitness

Aerobic fitness involves the functioning of your heart, lungs, and cardiovascular system. Aerobic exercises make your heart work harder, speeding up your heart rate and sending more richly oxygenated blood coursing through your circulatory system to feed all of the tissues of your body. Aerobic exercise has a number of benefits:

- It builds strong, healthy heart muscle.
- It increases the capacity of your lungs, so you don't get short of breath.
- It helps your body regulate cholesterol levels and keep arterial walls clean and wide.
- It builds your muscle endurance and improves muscle strength.
- It burns calories and body fat.
- It builds resistance to disease, including diabetes, cancer, high blood pressure, and heart disease.

Aerobic exercises offer weight-training benefits when your body is upright and your muscles have to support its weight through the exercise movements. Aerobic exercises that include a weight-bearing component such as jogging, walking, step-training, dance aerobics, kick-boxing, and skiing help build strong bones and prevent the development of osteoporosis.

Though your health care provider or fitness consultant will help you determine your specific goals, aerobic exercise is effective when it raises your resting heart rate—your normal heart rate during a period of inactivity—to a target heart rate, which is approximately 60 to 75 percent of your maximum heart rate. A treadmill or other fitness test can determine your maximum and target heart rates, but here is a general formula for finding a target heart rate (your health care provider can help you determine your individual numbers):

1. Subtract your age from 220 to find an approximate maximum heart rate.
2. Multiply that number by 60 percent; the result is your low-end target heart rate.

3. Multiply the maximum heart rate number from step 1 by 75 percent; the result is your high-end target heart rate.

You can gauge how well your exercise has helped you achieve your target heart rate by taking your pulse immediately after exercising. Take your pulse and count the number of heartbeats per fifteen seconds, then multiply that by four to get the number of beats per minute; then see how the result compares to your target heart rate numbers.

Any activity that gets your heart rate up and sustains it for fifteen to thirty minutes is an aerobic exercise; this category includes brisk walking, jogging, swimming, skiing, dancing, bicycling, rowing, hiking, rock climbing, stair climbing, cardio-boxing, power yoga, and a host of other movement-related activities. Most health and fitness experts recommend that you get at least a moderate amount of aerobic activity every day—forty-five minutes to an hour is great. You can break the activity up into smaller chunks of time, if that works better for you. So, on workdays, you could spend ten minutes on a stationary bike in the morning, take a ten-minute walk after lunch, and do a fifteen or twenty-minute video workout at home before dinner. On the weekend, you might substitute an hour-long bike ride, a forty-minute hike in a nearby park, or an hour of swimming laps. If you can't do aerobic exercises every day, try to do them at least four days a week, even if it doesn't add up to forty-five minutes each and every time.

The benefits of aerobic exercise are many, but they aren't permanent. To maintain your aerobic fitness, you have to keep up your aerobic exercise—and vary the specific type, frequency, and intensity of that exercise from time to time. Your body needs continued challenges to remain fit.

The choices are many, but variety is an important key when planning a successful aerobic exercise plan. Regular exercise is important, but variety within your schedule is crucial. Don't develop an everyday routine that involves the same walk, the same bike ride, or the same dance routine. Changing things around from time to time continually challenges your body's muscles to meet new demands and make new improvements. Variety helps you avoid becoming bored with your exercise plan. (If you're bored with your exercise routine, you're likely to drop it.)

Some sources estimate that approximately 60 percent of people who begin an exercise program drop it within the first six months. Your commitment to exercise has to last a lifetime, so make it a work in progress by continually evaluating and adapting it to match your growing fitness capabilities, interests, and needs.

ESSENTIALS

Whatever type of aerobic exercise you choose, always precede your workout with a five-minute period of stretching and a gradual warmup toward your full-force aerobic work. At the end of your exercise, spend another five minutes gradually cooling off with, for example, some slow walking or a series of deep-breathing exercises and long, slow stretches.

Strength Exercises

Strength training used to be considered the pastime of health-club hulks and muscle-men. Not any more; health experts today recommend weight training as an important component of the exercise program for all people, of all ages. Strength training involves performing a series of repetitive, weight-bearing motions, usually using free weights or some other means of providing resistance against the actions of your muscles. Fixed weight machines, such as the Nautilus line, are available at most gyms and health clubs. Floor work exercises, such as push-ups and sit-ups, some yoga postures and certain Pilate's matwork exercises, also provide resistance training benefits for building strength.

And the benefits of strength building are many. Strength training improves your muscular strength and endurance, of course, but it also helps improve the health and mobility of your joints. Strength training aids balance and coordination, and it builds strong bones—an especially important benefit for women in perimenopause or menopause. People of any age benefit from strength training; many assisted living and convalescent centers incorporate strength-training exercises in daily routines for even their bed- or wheelchair-bound residents.

You have a number of options for incorporating strength-training activities into your exercise program. Gym equipment such as most Nautilus-type machines offer a great way to ease into resistance training. These machines have adjustable weight levels, and most help you position your body properly to perform the exercises safely and get the maximum benefit from your weight lifting action. A fitness instructor can help you construct an exercise program that includes the use of these machines.

If you have a fever or are recovering from a severe illness, don't push yourself to maintain your regular exercise routine; gradually return to your exercise program as you recover. It's rarely a good idea to work through the burn; if any exercise feels painful or exhausting, reduce the weight you're lifting, do fewer repetitions, or slow down.

You don't need to join a gym or buy expensive equipment to get a good strength-training workout. You can buy a set of inexpensive free weights to do arm curls and lifts at home. (You can even lift cans of soup.) You can strap on arm and ankle weights while you clean the house or take your daily walk. You can create a floor-work exercise routine that incorporates traditional exercises such as sit-ups, push-ups, leg lifts, and "air bicycling." Or, you can buy a home-workout video that demonstrates yoga postures, t'ai chi exercises, Pilates movements, or other types of programs that include weight-bearing or resistance-training benefits.

In general, you perform weight-training exercises in sets of repetitions. Though your health care or fitness professional will help you design a program that's right for you, most people begin weight lifting, for example, with a weight they can lift six or eight times. (Each lift is a repetition.) You may begin by performing two or three sets of six or eight repetitions, then gradually increase the number of repetitions and the amount of the weight over time. In general, people who want to lose weight but gain muscle tone should do more repetitions using less heavy weights; people who want to increase strength dramatically and bulk up should exercise with heavier weights but do fewer repetitions.

Most medical and fitness experts agree that strength training should make up a smaller portion of your total weekly fitness plan than your aerobic training. Your health professional will help you determine how much (and what kind) of weight-training work is right for you. But in general, you may want to include at least one hour of total weight-training time in your weekly schedule. You can divide that time up into smaller segments, working fifteen minutes a day, four days a week, if that schedule fits your routine.

Strength training works to improve both muscle strength and endurance. The amount of resistance (or the weight you lift or push against) provides the strength-building function of weight training. You build endurance through continued resistance—increasing the total number of repetitions in each workout.

Flexibility Training

Your flexibility is determined by the length, strength, and elasticity of your muscles and the range of motion of your joints. Your range of motion may be different from anyone else's—your joints are unique in their intricate makeup and conformation. But your movement patterns and lifestyle habits can determine whether you can achieve the full range of motion your joints are physically capable of or whether you become stiff and inflexible.

Joints require movement and use in order to remain flexible and functional. Movement helps increase the elasticity of muscles and tendons, and it helps stimulate the circulation of blood through the tissues of the joint to keep them well-nourished and healthy. Long periods of inactivity allow muscles and tendons to grow stiff; when that happens, your range of motion shrinks, and movements can become awkward and painful.

Flexibility is an important quality for any active life. Every time you need to stoop to pick up a child, turn around to lift something from the backseat of the car, or reach up to place canned goods on the top shelf of your cabinet, you call upon your ability to stretch your muscles and flex your joints. Most sports, such as tennis, golf, and racquet ball, demand strong, flexible muscles and joints. And flexibility contributes to good balance and coordination; if you slip on a wet floor or stumble over an obstacle in the dark, your flexibility may determine your ability to recover your balance and avoid a fall. If you do fall, you'll suffer less injury and recover more quickly if your body is flexible and strong.

FACTS

Obesity contributes to osteoarthritis by putting an excessive load on weight-bearing joints (such as the hip and knee). If you have this form of arthritis, however, your doctor will encourage you to exercise, both to help reduce your weight and rehabilitate damaged joints. A rehabilitation therapist can design an exercise program for your specific needs.

Stretching is an important exercise for increasing flexibility. Remember, you should begin and end every exercise session with at least five minutes of stretching and warmup movements. Many exercise practices and programs, including yoga and Pilates, incorporate stretching into most of their exercise movements. Flexibility training typically focuses on shoulders, hips, knees, and the hamstrings (muscles that extend up the back of your thighs). Stretches are slow, controlled movements that gently lengthen and tone the muscles and flex the joints, to give them increased elasticity and strength.

Choosing an Exercise Program

You have a number of options for pulling together a sensible, effective exercise program that will give you the aerobic, strengthening, and flexibility training you need. It's important that the program meet your physical and emotional needs. You need to enjoy the time you spend exercising; otherwise, you're likely to lose interest in it after a short period of time. The following are some issues to consider.

- **Are you better suited to working out alone or are you motivated by working in a group?**
- **How much assistance will you need to begin your program?** You may prefer to begin with the on-site advice of a fitness instructor in a gym, then do more of your work on your own.
- **Can you incorporate both indoor and outdoor exercises into your routine?** Designing an exercise plan that involves as much variety as possible is one way to make sure you'll remain interested and engaged in it.
- **How much money are you willing to spend on gym fees and equipment?** If you sign up for an expensive exercise program, the cost could become a reason to drop it after a short time. Look for seasonal price specials or introductory programs if price could become an issue for you.
- **Will the program you've chosen be convenient—or even doable—given your schedule?** If you choose a gym or workout center that's across town from your home and job, you'll be tempted to skip it more often. If you have to drag out heavy equipment or chase the rest of your family away from the television in order to work out, it may not take long before you decide it isn't worth the effort.
- **Does your program incorporate exercises that will help you build strength, aerobic endurance, and flexibility?** Don't create a program that's going to box you in to any one type of exercise or a single routine. By varying the type, intensity, and length of exercises within your program, you'll continue to challenge your body as its capabilities improve over time.

Be open to suggestions and be creative. Hang around with your kids and play catch. Go for a long walk after dinner with a special friend or by yourself. Lift telephone books while you're on the phone. Put on your favorite dance music and hop around while you fold laundry. It's all about getting off your fanny and getting the blood moving again, any way you can. Every calorie you burn, every muscle you flex, every joint you move, is a point in your favor. The more you do, the faster those points add up.

Don't give up. Even if you have to step away from your usual exercise routine for a few weeks due to work or illness, get back into it as soon as time and circumstances permit. And don't let weight gain embarrass you into staying away from the gym. You're taking a positive step toward improving your physical condition, and that's something to be proud of. Changes for the positive will be gradual, so don't be disappointed if the miracle transformation doesn't happen overnight. Keep at it, and you'll see the results.

QUESTIONS?

I want a program I can commit to; what's a good way to start?
Walking has the lowest dropout rate of any exercise program. It's free, you don't need a lot of special equipment, and you can do it throughout your life. Most experts recommend walking more than three miles per hour if you're walking for weight loss. (You burn 416 calories per hour at that speed.) But don't forget to mix it up, and add other activities to build a complete exercise program.

CHAPTER 15

Taking Care of All of You

The wide range of physical and emotional changes that may accompany perimenopause and menopause puts demands on your body and mind that you've probably never experienced before. Paying extra attention to a few body care basics can help minimize the effects of aging and keep you feeling fit and refreshed through your busy days and nights.

Appreciating the Woman in the Mirror

As you read about menopause and the special health concerns that accompany the aging process, you might start to feel like your body is simply a collection of potential problems that need constant monitoring and cautious attention. It's true that the human body becomes more susceptible to certain diseases and conditions with age and that women face special health concerns as their natural hormone supply diminishes in menopause. But you are more than a pair of breasts, a uterus, a heart, and a set of bones; you're a woman, with a life full of interests that extend well beyond disease prevention.

Every woman expects the natural changes of age to occur, but in a culture that seems to worship the physical impossibilities of eternal youth, rail-like thinness, and nonstop sexual vigor and allure, maintaining an appreciation and respect for your body as it ages can be difficult. One of the benefits of maturity is a growing appreciation for the valuable things pop culture often fails to acknowledge. If you continue to evaluate your appearance and physical capabilities in comparison to those of a twenty-year-old, you're destined to be dissatisfied and disappointed.

FACTS

According to the National Center for Health Statistics, the average woman in the United States over the age of twenty is just under 5'4" tall and weighs 152 pounds. Some studies of women in the fashion industry reveal that the average fashion model is 5'11" tall and weighs 117 pounds. You can decide for yourself which of these is more realistic.

The surest way to look your best is to acknowledge and appreciate the woman you are now. Then, focus your attention on keeping that woman as healthy and happy as you possibly can. If you feel better, you will look better. Eat the foods that are right for you, follow the exercise program you need, keep every one of your annual health-maintenance checkups, give your skin and hair the extra care it needs, and pamper yourself with the extra rest and relaxation you deserve. Taking good care of the woman you are today is the first and most important secret to looking and feeling your best through menopause and beyond. And part of that whole woman maintenance plan involves taking good care of your eyes, ears, and teeth.

You depend upon your senses to remain in communication with the world around you, and good eyesight and hearing are essential to that dialog. Though few women need to worry about experiencing a rapid decline in the quality of their vision or hearing as they near the age of menopause, those functions can begin to diminish around the age of forty or fifty. Some of the physical changes of menopause can have an impact on the health of your teeth, as well. Though age-related changes are inevitable, you can minimize their impact by taking special care of your teeth, eyes, and ears; by watching for signs and symptoms of potential problems; and by incorporating regular checkups into your regular health care routine.

SSENTIALS Some medications can change your vision, either by reducing your ability to focus or by reducing your eyes' lubrication, making them dry and itchy. If you notice changes in your vision shortly after you've begun taking a new medication, contact the doctor who prescribed the medication and report the change immediately.

Monitoring Changes in Vision

Around the age of forty, many women begin to experience ocular problems, otherwise known as changes in vision. The shape of your eyeball can change as you age, and the subsequent reduction of your visual acuity can be subtle at first. A few of the most common problems you might encounter after age forty include:

- You may develop problems reading small print or seeing objects clearly that are close to your eyes. This condition is known as presbyopia, and usually is easy to correct with reading glasses, or even over-the-counter magnifying glasses from the drugstore.

- You might begin to notice tiny specks or odd dust-like particles passing before your vision. These "floaters" usually are just a normal condition of the aging eye. If they become extreme in number, or are accompanied by bright flashes of light, you should contact your ophthalmologist immediately. A sudden increase in the numbers of floaters can be a warning of a retinal tear or other more serious vision problem.
- You may experience problems with your eyes becoming dry and irritated after you spend some time reading or working at the computer. Again, this problem isn't unusual in overforty eyes, and you may be able to alleviate it by using "artificial tears" (available over the counter in most drugstores) for better lubrication.

ALERT

If you work at a computer, don't allow your eyes to focus for long periods of time on the screen. Look up and away from your computer screen every fifteen minutes or so, and don't forget to blink now and then. Overuse and strain can take a toll on eyes, and long, uninterrupted hours at the computer can contribute to the damage.

Pay attention to your vision; don't ignore developing problems. Some people experience a substantial loss in the quality of their vision before they realize that the problem even exists. That's why all women (and men for that matter) after the age of forty should get regular annual eye examinations by an ophthalmologist. Women over the age of fifty are at particular risk of developing eye diseases, some of which might be connected to the loss of the body's natural estrogens. Your ophthalmologist will check for the following age-related diseases during your exam:

- Macular degeneration attacks the center of the retina, so central vision diminishes while peripheral vision remains unchanged. Macular degeneration can make reading and driving impossible; it's the number one cause of blindness in women age sixty-five and over. Macular degeneration is thought to be the most common reason for older people to fail their driver's license renewal exam—

they flunk the eye exam, not the written or driving parts of the test. No cure for the disease is known, but its risk factors include being menopausal or postmenopausal, a family history of the disease, smoking, perhaps high blood pressure, and overexposure to the sun and other ultraviolet (UV) rays. Some studies, such as the Beaver Dam Study, suggested that estrogen replacement helps postpone or prevent the onset of macular degeneration; talk to your doctor for more information.

- Glaucoma damages the optic nerve and is caused by a buildup of fluid, and thus pressure, inside the eye. When doctors detect and treat glaucoma early, the eye can escape permanent nerve damage. Chronic glaucoma develops slowly and, in most cases, is only detectable in its early stage through an eye examination. Acute glaucoma can happen suddenly, blurring the vision and causing a number of symptoms including nausea and dizziness. Risk factors include being over forty, being African American, having a family history of glaucoma, having diabetes, or being nearsighted.

FACTS

Doctors can't reverse the optic nerve damage caused by glaucoma, so early detection is essential. Ophthalmologists can test for glaucoma using a number of procedures. The simplest of these tests involves applying a short burst of air to your eye and determining how the surface of the eye responds to the pressure.

Your best prescription for maintaining good eye health after age forty includes:

- Getting regular annual eye examinations by an ophthalmologist.
- Eating a healthy diet, including your full daily nutritional requirements. (See Chapter 14.)
- Noticing and reporting to your doctor or ophthalmologist vision changes such as reduced night vision, clouded or blurry vision, bright flashes in your peripheral vision, or changes in your perception of color.
- Wearing good UV-resistant eye protection while outdoors.

Protecting Your Hearing

After age fifty, many women experience some hearing loss and by age sixty-five, nearly one-third of all women have some decline in hearing. You might not be aware that your hearing is fading until someone you live or work with brings it to your attention. Most age-related hearing loss is gradual and can develop slowly over a period of years.

Some types of hearing loss can be the result of a physical injury, an infection, medication, or the development of growths or tumors. These hearing losses are called sensorineural (caused by damage to the nerves that transmit sound from the ear to the brain), because the sensors in the inner ear lose their ability to send sound signals to the brain. Long-term exposure to loud noise causes this type of hearing loss, so if you spent the 1960s with your ears glued to the loud speakers at rock concerts, you could experience this type of hearing loss.

FACTS

Working near loud machinery, including lawn mowers and leaf blowers, can cause serious harm to your hearing. Avoid loud noise when you can. When you can't avoid the noise, wear earplugs or protective headphones. You may feel like an old fogey when you move to the back of the rock concert crowd, but there's nothing young and sexy about losing your hearing.

Conductive hearing loss occurs when sounds don't reach your inner ear properly, due to problems with something other than the transmitting nerves themselves. If you have a history of ear infections, damage to your eardrum, or even accumulations of earwax within your ear canal, you can experience this type of hearing loss. And, as the tissue within the ear canal becomes thinner and drier, it becomes less effective at transmitting sound.

Regular hearing checkups can reveal either type of hearing damage, but you also need to pay attention to changes in your hearing. If you notice that you're turning the television up louder these days or constantly asking people to repeat what they've just said to you, you're probably experiencing some hearing damage. Losing your hearing can make you feel isolated and out of touch with the world around you. Take steps to protect your ears and monitor changes, so you can correct developing problems before they become irreversible.

Keeping Teeth Healthy

You know about the importance of regular dental checkups, brushing, and flossing. And you also know that maintaining a healthy diet that includes a wide variety of fruit, vegetables, whole grains, and necessary vitamin and mineral supplements is an essential part of maintaining full physical health, including healthy teeth and gums. But did you know that menopause can present some special challenges to your dental health? As your body's natural estrogen supply diminishes in menopause, your gum tissues can become thinner and less elastic, and bone loss can contribute to the development of gingivitis and periodontitis—gum diseases in which the soft tissue of the jaw deteriorates around the roots of the teeth.

If the bone density of the jaw itself diminishes, the socket of the tooth loosens its grip, and tooth loss can result. Osteoporosis in the rest of the body can be a silent process, but greater numbers of dentists are noticing loose teeth in their menopausal patients as the first overt sign of decreasing bone density in the body overall.

If you've slacked off in some of your dental maintenance measures in the past, you have to get over that tendency now. Healthy teeth and gums will help keep you feeling vital and fit and looking your best. Bad dental health habits can catch up with you as you move into your postmenopausal years. Some estimates show that over one-third of all women over the age of sixty have lost most or all of their teeth. To avoid joining that group, here's a simple plan for maintaining your dental health after forty:

- See your dentist twice a year for checkups and cleaning.
- Brush your teeth at least twice a day; use a soft toothbrush and floss afterward. Brush for two to five minutes, morning and evening (a third cleaning after lunch would be even better)—according to the Chicago Dental Society, it takes at least two minutes of brushing to remove plaque and bacteria.

- Make sure you're getting enough calcium in your diet, and limit the amount of sugar you consume.
- Pay special attention to signs of gum disease, such as bleeding or inflamed gums.
- Drink plenty of water—thirty-two to sixty-four ounces every day. Water is essential for hydrating your system. It can help rinse bacteria from your gum tissue and keep the tissue moist and healthy.

Those "water spray" tooth cleaners aren't as effective as a soft-bristle toothbrush and dental floss at removing tartar and plaque buildup between teeth—the number one cause of gingivitis. Plaque-removing mouthwashes can help soften and loosen plaque. Take the time to clean your teeth right to avoid the pain (and potential tooth loss) of gum disease.

If you have the time to floss only once a day, do it at night, right before you go to sleep. That's also a good time to use antiplaque or fluoride rinses; you'll have a six- to eight-hour period without eating or drinking, so you can absorb protective fluoride and antibacterial agents.

Caring for Your Skin and Hair

If you have had no other signs of the passing years, you're likely to see some changes reflected in your hair and skin. As skin ages it loses elasticity and becomes thinner, drier, and more prone to itching and sagging. Your hair becomes thinner, too; it breaks more easily and grows in more slowly. Some of these changes are due to the body's diminishing levels of estrogen. Estrogen helps keep healthy tissues well nourished and moisturized; without it, both skin and hair lose strength and elasticity and grow thinner. Other changes are the result of age; as you grow older, your body slows in its production of new cells and collagen production slows. Collagen is the basic bridgework, or support system, for all the fibrous tissue of your body, of which skin is only one component. Normal collagen helps keep the skin plump and resilient, providing part of the skin's support structure. Taking estrogen helps maintain the proper collagen content in tissues throughout your body.

FACTS

The fluctuations in hormone levels you experience during perimenopause and menopause can result in a relative increase in androgen levels as compared to estrogen levels. As androgen levels rise, facial hairs can become thicker, darker, more numerous, and more noticeable. Rogue chin hairs are a common occurrence for women age forty and over.

Exposure to the sun is another culprit in the deterioration of your skin's elasticity and moisture. The ultraviolet rays of the sun begin damaging the skin of young children; as sun exposure builds over the years, the damage becomes increasingly severe and apparent. Proper use of sunscreen with enough UV protection (SPF 15 or higher) and using hats or caps and sunglasses to shade your face and eyes may delay or prevent this damage.

Skin Care Basics

Your diet, the amount of rest you get every day, the level of stress you're subjected to, and the types of pollutants that exist in your environment all play a role in the health and vitality of your skin. Women in the United States spend millions of dollars every year on skin-rejuvenating treatments, including:

- Chemical peels and dermabrasion treatments that remove the outer layers of the skin
- Injections of botulinum toxin (bo-tox) that temporarily paralyze the facial muscles to eliminate frown lines and other wrinkles in the face and neck
- Collagen injections that temporarily plump up the skin's understructure
- Cosmetic surgery that tightens, tucks, and lifts skin to eliminate wrinkling and sagging

All of these treatment options can improve the appearance of aging skin, but some of those improvements are expensive and temporary. And— as with any medical treatment—all of these techniques carry some risks, which are infrequent, but include scarring and skin discoloration. Carefully research any treatment option you're considering by getting multiple professional opinions and by talking to others who have used the procedure.

FACTS

Don't rely on magazine articles, a facialist, or a cosmetic salesperson for skin care advice. Talk to a plastic surgeon or a dermatologist about your skin concerns. He or she can help you pinpoint specific skin problems you might be developing and tell you the best techniques for combating them.

If you prefer to pursue less invasive techniques for keeping your skin looking healthy and vital, you have many options to choose from. Though your skin is unique, most women need to moisturize their skin more frequently after age forty. A number of creams, lotions, and even some prescription drugs are available today for nourishing and healing aging skin:

- Creams and lotions containing alpha hydroxy acids (AHAs) dissolve the upper layer of skin that has suffered the most damage to reveal fresher, plumper skin beneath. These products won't eliminate deep wrinkles or age spots, but they can make the skin look and feel fresher. Some women experience skin rashes and irritations when using these creams and lotions. Women with sensitive skin or rosacea should not use these products without the advice of a health care professional.
- Oils, creams, and lotions containing antioxidants and vitamin derivatives may help protect collagen, moisturize the skin's upper layer, and help diminish the visible signs of fine wrinkles. Vitamins C, E, and A are typical antioxidants used in these products. Some women report that their skin looks younger and fresher with the regular use of these products, but results vary.

- Retinol, a vitamin A derivative, is also a common antiaging formula component. Prescription drugs Retin-A and Renova are marketed to reduce fine-line wrinkles, build collagen, and help fade age spots. As with other skin care products, some women report that these drugs help their skin look younger and fresher, but results vary. Talk to your dermatologist to learn more.

Beyond skin care formulas, however, you have some very basic tools at your disposal for protecting your skin. No matter what other skin care treatments you use, follow these basic practices to protect your skin and keep it looking its best:

- Drink at least thirty-two ounces of water every day—sixty-four ounces is better.
- Stop smoking—smoking ages the skin, breaks down its collagen structure, and increases wrinkles and sagging, especially around the mouth and the eyes.
- Anytime you go outdoors, use a sunscreen with an SPF of 15 or higher, even if skies are overcast.
- Maintain a daily skin care routine of gentle washing in lukewarm water, using a very mild soap. Avoid soaps with excessive perfumes and deodorizing chemicals, and don't scrub your skin! Use a moisturizer everywhere your skin feels dry, but especially around your eyes, mouth, throat, and hands.

Keeping Your Hair Healthy and Strong

The changes in your hair growth and health in perimenopause and postmenopause can seem downright unfair; the hair on your scalp starts to become thin, sparse, and grey, while some of the previously fine, pale hairs on your face grow thicker and darker. You can tweeze, wax, or chemically dissolve unwanted facial hair, or use electrolysis to permanently destroy the hair follicle. (Some women experience skin irritation from electrolysis.) Though some of these changes are inevitable with age, you have a number of options available to you for preserving the health and vitality of your hair.

First, the basics: Keep your hair trimmed to remove split, brittle ends and encourage volume. Some color treatments can give the effect of fullness and volumizing shampoos can coat thin hair to give it extra body. When you shampoo, use warm—not hot—water, and limit blow-drying as much as possible. Some deep conditioning treatments, used every few weeks, can help keep hair strong and less prone to breaking and splitting.

Your hair reflects your nutrition, too. Don't forget to include a wide variety of fresh fruit and vegetables in your diet, and take vitamin supplements to make sure that you're getting all of the recommended nutrients every day. Proper hydration is essential to healthy hair, so don't forget to drink the recommended thirty-two ounces or more of water every day.

Some prescription drugs are available to help manage menopausal hair problems:

- Minoxidil (marketed under the name Rogaine) works to stimulate hair follicles that may have grown dormant. Minoxidil can help restore lost hair by 10 percent or more, according to some estimates.
- Eflornithine may help stop unwanted hair growth. Eflornithine (marketed in its topical form as Vaniqa) can be applied as a cream directly to the area where unwanted hair growth occurs. The drug inhibits the production of an enzyme that contributes to hair growth; as a result, the drug slows the growth of unwanted hair.

Thinning, dry, brittle hair may be more than a natural sign of age. Some medications and certain systemic illnesses, such as a thyroid disorder, can also cause hair to lose its strength and vitality—even to the point of causing dramatic hair loss. Talk to your doctor or health care provider about noticeable changes to your hair's strength and appearance; don't assume you're just looking your age.

These hair and skin preparations and prescriptions take weeks, if not months, to show a result. Don't be discouraged and give up your treatment program if you don't see results overnight.

Making Time for Rest and Relaxation

Stress and fatigue are the enemies of your health, vitality, and natural beauty. Many of the most common symptoms of perimenopause and menopause, including mood swings, hot flashes, headaches, high blood pressure, and lethargy, are caused or complicated by excess stress and lack of rest. You may be accustomed to thinking of your body as a nonstop powerhouse that thrives on stress and performs best under pressure. Even if that belief held true when you were twenty, it doesn't hold true now. Your body and mind need adequate amounts of rest and enjoyment, especially during the years preceding menopause.

FACTS

If you don't find positive ways to relax and reduce stress, you'll probably find negative ways to do so. Many people turn to food, alcohol, or drugs to help ease stress or avoid feelings of low self-esteem, anxiety, or boredom. When you feel that taking time for leisure and relaxation is an indulgence, think about the potential

Participating in regular aerobic and strengthening exercise is critical for maintaining your body's ability to enjoy healthy, restful sleep. But part of your weekly fitness plan should also include some time—every day—for relaxation. Even thirty minutes of planned relaxation a day can make a big difference in your physical and mental health. Determine what relaxation technique works best for you—many activities can soothe your mind and rejuvenate feelings of well-being. Here are just a few suggestions:

- Mind/body practices, such as relaxation exercises, meditation, yoga, or t'ai chi (see Chapter 14)
- Reading, listening to music, or playing an instrument
- Talking with friends, spending time with your partner, playing catch with your children, walking your dog
- Soaking your feet, taking a leisurely bath, or giving yourself a facial
- Gardening, painting, writing in a journal
- Reading religious texts or practicing your faith

If your life is crowded, busy, and packed with a long to-do list of weighty responsibilities, you may need to force yourself to sit back, relax, and enjoy life for a few moments every day. But you'll do yourself and your family, job, and friends a favor by keeping your body and mind well rested and relaxed. You won't look good, feel good, or perform well if you starve yourself of leisure. As you move through menopause, you have to consider rest and relaxation an essential luxury for a physically and emotionally healthy life.

Stress can lead to insomnia and the long list of health problems associated with a lack of healthy, restful sleep. For important information on how to promote good sleep, see Chapter 10, "Your Mind, Mood, and Emotional Health."

CHAPTER 16

Coping with Hot Flashes

When women seek relief of menopause symptoms, hot flashes are the symptom they cite most often. Though hot flashes fade over time, severe vasomotor symptoms can disrupt both the waking and sleeping hours of your busy life for several years. Fortunately, you have many options to choose from for reducing or eliminating hot flashes, but you need to choose carefully—and in consultation with your health care professional.

A Short Review of the Hot Flash Facts

Nearly 90 percent of all women passing through the stages of menopause will experience hot flashes during some part of the transition. Though hot flashes are a common symptom of menopause, in many cases they are minor inconveniences rather than alarming problems. Hot flashes (sometimes called hot flushes) typically begin with an increase in heart rate and a slight feeling of warmth, usually occurring in the face, neck, and shoulders. Women describe hot flashes differently, depending upon the frequency and severity of their own experience.

Mild or moderate hot flashes may last anywhere from one to fifteen minutes, and cause feelings of mild warmth, accompanied by light perspiration and a slightly dry mouth. After the flash passes, the skin may feel slightly clammy. Mild hot flashes pass with little or no impact on general feelings of well-being.

FACTS

Most women begin having hot flashes within the first year after they stop menstruating. Women who undergo induced or surgical menopause are most prone to suffering hot flashes. The immediate drop in hormone production that follows removal of the ovaries or a temporary interruption in their functions can result in sudden and severe vasomotor symptoms.

Severe hot flashes can last up to forty-five minutes, and cause the skin temperature to rise dramatically. The face, neck, and throat can become flushed and red and the body can break out in heavy perspiration. A woman experiencing a severe hot flash can have difficulty breathing, and the hot flash can induce panic attacks and distress. Afterward, the woman may be left with a headache, some nausea, and a general feeling of anxiety and exhaustion.

If hot flashes are severe or long-lasting, they can contribute to a number of issues that can have a negative effect on your health and well-being. Hot flashes that occur at night—often known as night sweats—can interrupt sleep and lead to daytime fatigue, exhaustion, and decreased cognitive abilities.

The fear of breaking into a clothes-drenching sweat during business meetings or social events can lead to anxiety and even depression.

When hot flashes degrade the quality of your sleep or prevent you from being fully functional during the day, you need to take action. Some of the most widely recommended and effective methods for easing or eliminating the frequency and severity of these symptoms are discussed later in this chapter.

What's Happening When You Have a Hot Flash?

Hot flashes are connected to changes in your estrogen levels, though the specific cause and effect relationship is still under study. Though flagging levels of estrogen may set the stage for hot flashes, the actual hot flashes are the result of a sudden resetting of the body's thermostat. If your brain senses that your body is too hot—for any reason, including low estrogen, increased blood flow to the brain, a high ambient temperature, or even the ingestion of hot, spicy foods—it sends out a signal that your body needs to cool off. In response, your pituitary gland sends out luteinizing hormone (LH), which causes the blood vessels near your skin's surface to dilate to release heat through your skin. This heat-releasing action makes your skin temperature (and your body temperature) rise, followed by an increase in perspiration. The perspiration helps to cool the skin, which can result in a clammy feeling. If you've perspired heavily, you may be left damp and even chilly. Your body temperature drops and your blood vessels constrict. If you are damp and cold, you may begin to shiver. That's the hot flash in action.

If you suffer from severe hot flashes, it's not unusual to have feelings of nausea, headache, and weakness afterward—especially when hot flashes last for thirty or forty-five minutes. If your feelings of intense heat last for longer than an hour, you may not be experiencing symptoms of perimenopause or menopause, and you should consult your doctor or other health care professional.

Common Hot Flash Triggers

As mentioned, hot flashes are signals that your body may be suffering fluctuating levels of estrogen or that your estrogen levels have declined dramatically. But other factors can cause hot flashes or contribute to their severity. Many women find, for example, that they have hot flashes during periods of anxiety and nervousness; other studies have found that some prescription antihypertensive and antianxiety medications may also cause hot flashes. As mentioned earlier, hot flashes may indicate that your body is reacting to certain foods or beverages or even the temperature of the air around you—some women report their hot flashes are more severe and last longer when they occur during hot weather or in a hot room.

How Many, How Bad, How Long?

Although many women don't seem to notice hot flashes until after menopause has occurred, many others begin having them during perimenopause, with forty-eight being an average age for the onset of hot flashes.

A number of studies have been conducted on the prevalence, frequency, and intensity of hot flashes in perimenopausal and menopausal women. In general, women who experience hot flashes start having them within at least one year before menopause, and continue having them for one to six years.

The American College of Obstetricians and Gynecologists's publication *Managing Menopause* lists the findings of one study, in which 501 women were asked about the frequency and severity of their hot flashes. Of those participating in the study, 87 percent reported having one or more flashes per day; of those experiencing multiple daily hot flashes, the numbers of incidents per day ranged from five to fifty, with one-third of the women reporting more than ten. Another study reported a lower frequency of hot flashes—participants had an average of only three or four flashes a day. That study also showed that, on average, hot flashes lasted about three and one-half minutes, though some can come and go in no more than five seconds. And in nearly every study, almost three-fourths of the respondents said their hot flashes were mild, moderate, or only variably intense.

Techniques for Turning Down the Heat

A number of treatment options to help you alleviate—or even eliminate—hot flashes caused by the onset of menopause are discussed later in this chapter. But you have a variety of first-defense techniques available to you that don't require any special medication or therapeutic program. Try these simple techniques to avoid hot flashes or minimize their severity:

- **Avoid triggering foods and drinks.** Spicy foods—foods heavy in capsaicin, the heat-inducing chemical in cayenne and other hot peppers—can contribute to hot flashes. Caffeine and alcohol are also common triggers, so you should avoid caffeinated beverages, excessive amounts of chocolate, and alcoholic beverages if you are suffering from hot flashes.

- **Drink plenty of water during the day—at least thirty-two ounces, more if possible.** Keep a glass of ice water with you during meetings and conferences and set a thermal-lined drink container of ice water on your nightstand, ready to help cool down raging hot flashes.

- **Get at least thirty minutes of exercise every day.** Regular exercise is an integral part of any healthy lifestyle, but it might offer specific relief from vasomotor symptoms. Exercise, including stretching, aerobic, and weight-bearing activities, has been shown to cut down on the frequency of hot flashes, and may even help limit the length and severity of hot flashes that occur. Regular exercise also promotes a general feeling of well-being that can help reduce anxiety and stress that can contribute to hot flashes.

- **Wear layers of moisture-absorbing clothing.** When a hot flash strikes, you can take off one or more layers of clothing to help cool your skin temperature quickly. Cotton fabrics are particularly helpful in allowing adequate air to reach the skin, and they're good at absorbing perspiration. Cotton wicks moisture away from the skin and into the air, so both you and your clothing can dry more quickly. Tightly woven synthetic fabrics can hold in both body heat and moisture, making the hot flash more severe and its effects more long lasting.

- **Keep your thermostat turned down—seventy degrees or lower during the day, and sixty-five degrees or lower at night.** Lower temperatures can help ward off the onset of hot flashes, and you'll cool off more quickly from those that do occur when the air around you is cool. Keep a fan handy, and turn it on whenever necessary. If you suffer from night sweats, it's especially important that you keep your bedroom temperature cool; don't skimp on the air conditioning, and use a fan to keep the air moving around your room.

- **Manage stress to the best of your ability.** Avoid stress if you can, but be prepared for stressful situations you can't sidestep. Deep breathing exercises, meditation, yoga, and visualization are all helpful techniques for boosting your ability to remain calm and centered throughout your day. Massage therapy and acupressure can also help you manage your response to stress and reduce the frequency of stress-induced hot flashes.

SSENTIALS

If a hot flash strikes, you may get some quick relief by running cold water over your hands, wrists, and inner elbow. A cold cloth on your forehead or the back of your neck can help, too; if you're at home, step into a cold shower and let the water run over you until the heat wave passes.

Hormonal Treatments for Hot Flash Relief

Though medical science continues to study the connection between hormone depletion and hot flashes, hormone replacement treatment—involving estrogen and/or progesterone—is the most effective medical treatment for vasomotor symptoms known today. According to the American College of Obstetricians and Gynecologists, 80 to 90 percent of women taking prescribed estrogen find relief from hot flashes.

Estrogen offers a number of other health benefits for women experiencing symptoms of perimenopause and menopause, including protection against osteoporosis and colorectal cancer. No other treatment for the relief of hot flashes offers the wide-ranging benefits of estrogen replacement therapy. Women using estrogen replacement for the treatment of hot flashes typically experience some relief within a few weeks of beginning treatment, though it may be a month or more before they begin to feel the maximum benefits of the estrogen treatment.

FACTS

Estrogen is a highly effective tool for combating symptoms of perimenopause and menopause, but it's not suitable for all women. See Chapter 11, "Understanding Hormones and HRT," for more information about the benefits and potential risks of estrogen.

Estrogen isn't recommended for women with a personal history of recently diagnosed endometrial cancer. For these women, progestins such as medroxyprogesterone or megestrol acetate, have been shown to offer relief from hot flashes. Some studies have shown progestins to decrease hot flashes by as much as 70 to 90 percent.

Another hormone-based treatment for hot flashes is progesterone cream. This cream, available through prescription, is rubbed on the skin, and the progesterone is slowly absorbed into the woman's system. Though some studies have shown that progesterone cream can offer significant relief from hot flashes, it can be accompanied by some negative side effects, including vaginal bleeding and PMS symptoms such as fatigue.

Only your doctor or health care professional can help you decide whether or not hormone-based treatments are your best choice for reducing or eliminating hot flashes. If you and your health care provider decide that hormones aren't right for you, you can choose from other treatment options, including other medications and hormone alternatives, discussed in the sections that follow.

Nonhormonal Medications

Though most medical experts prescribe some form of hormone therapy for the relief of vasomotor symptoms accompanying menopause, these treatments aren't appropriate for all women. Women with active endometrial or breast cancers, for example, usually must avoid hormone therapy during cancer treatment. Medical professionals rarely prescribe hormone therapy for women with a personal or family history of blood clotting, liver disease, or other conditions that can be triggered or exacerbated by hormone treatments. (See Chapter 11 for more information on hormone replacement therapy.)

To provide relief from hot flashes for women who cannot take estrogen, medical professionals can prescribe other medications that have been shown to offer some relief from hot flashes. The following list mentions some of these prescription medications for alleviating hot flashes:

- Clonidine hydrochloride reduces the responsiveness of the body's vascular system, and has been used for some time in the treatment of high blood pressure. A low dose is used; it may take three to four weeks to begin to see improvement in symptoms; blood pressure must also be monitored. Clonidine has some negative side effects, however; some tests have shown that Clonidine can disrupt the sleep of some women. Other side effects reported include dizziness and dry mouth.
- Methyldopa is another antihypertensive (high blood pressure medication) sometimes used to relieve vasomotor symptoms. Though methyldopa has been shown to reduce the number of hot flashes women experience during the day, it can cause dry mouth, dizziness, and headache.
- Selective serotonin reuptake inhibitors (SSRIs), including paroxetine and venlafaxine, are also used to lessen vasomotor symptoms, though doctors don't commonly prescribe them for that purpose. In higher doses, these drugs are used to treat depression. Some tests have shown that relatively low doses of these drugs can reduce the frequency and severity of hot flashes by as much as 50 to 75 percent, depending upon the specific drug and dosage strategy. Side effects of these drugs include dry mouth, nausea, and anxiety.
- Bellergal, a drug that combines very low dosages of belladonna and phenobarbital, is an FDA-approved medication for the treatment of menopausal symptoms. This drug has been used for decades in the short-term treatment of hot flashes, with varying success. Bellergal can have a number of unpleasant side effects, including constipation, dry mouth, and dizziness.

ESSENTIALS Many of the nonhormonal treatments for hot flashes and other menopause symptoms are controversial, and their effectiveness, safety, and possible side effects and interactions with other medications remain the subject of many ongoing studies.

Herbs, Botanicals, and Other Alternatives

You need to approach any alternative treatment option with open eyes and healthy skepticism. Botanical extracts, herbal supplements, and nutraceutical compounds aren't inspected or approved by the Food and Drug Administration, so they haven't passed the rigorous testing process of approved pharmaceuticals, and they haven't undergone a scientifically controlled process of long-term, in-depth study. Read Chapter 12, "Alternatives to Hormone Replacement Therapy," for a full discussion of this issue, and be aware that you can't just stroll down the aisle of your local health food store and choose a safe, effective, natural cure for any of your hormonal symptoms based on the claims of the label (or on other women's experiences you read about in popular consumer magazines or Internet chat rooms).

Doctors and scientists around the world, however, continue to evaluate the effectiveness of some of the most popular alternative treatments for the symptoms of menopause, because many women are choosing to use them. Nevertheless, a great deal remains to be learned about the safety, effectiveness, and long-term value of these treatment options.

Some of the alternative treatments most commonly used for the relief of hot flashes include:

- Soy products, including whole soy foods, soy protein capsules, and isoflavone extracts, offer some relief from mild hot flashes according to the results of a few studies. Soy proteins are available in soy milk, tofu, tempeh, and roasted soy nuts. Because researchers haven't determined how phytoestrogens in soy interact with cancerous cells, however, these products aren't recommended for women seeking nonhormonal relief from menopause symptoms due to a personal or family history of cancer. Many studies are under way on the use of soy in the treatment of menopause symptoms, so keep watching for new information, and ask your doctor about the latest developments.

- Some women have reported that taking vitamin E offered them relief from hot flashes. In studies where participants took a regulated daily dose of 800 international units of vitamin E, the women did experience some minor relief (on the order of one less hot flash per day), and the vitamin caused no negative side effects. Right now, no study supports the idea that you can achieve significant relief from hot flashes by taking vitamin E, but (again) studies continue in this area.

Research has not yet determined whether black cohosh is safe for women with breast cancer and other estrogen-sensitive cancers. If you suspect you may be pregnant, avoid taking black cohosh; it may cause miscarriage or premature birth.

- Black cohosh—derived from the root of an herb—is popular in Europe as a treatment for premenstrual syndrome and a number of menopausal symptoms. Though some products containing extracts of black cohosh carry labels that claim they can reduce hot flashes by as much as 25 percent, many medical experts feel that data to verify the herb's effectiveness is lacking. Black cohosh can have a number of negative side effects, including nausea and dizziness. When using black cohosh for the treatment of perimenopause or menopause symptoms, you should limit the total treatment time to no more than six months.

Mind-Body Exercises

Many women have found that they can limit the number and severity of hot flashes using mind-body practices such as yoga, meditation, visualization, and deep breathing. Stress, anxiety, and fatigue can contribute to the onset and severity of hot flashes; these techniques help calm the mind, relax your muscles and nerves, and keep you feeling rested and at ease. Even when hot flashes do occur, regular practice of these techniques can help you recover more quickly from their effects. And these relaxation techniques and mind-body exercises work to combat a number of other menopausal symptoms, including mood swings, sleeplessness, muscle loss, joint aches, and reduced cognitive functions.

ESSENTIALS

Use visualization techniques to help cool a hot flash before it builds to a three-alarm level. When you feel a hot flash begin to develop, close your eyes and envision being in a cool, breezy location. Think of the warmth as a liquid, and imagine that you can channel it to flow from your body. Envision the heat draining out through your hands and feet; as the heat leaves your body, imagine that a cool layer of snow is falling on your head, shoulders, and arms.

Use deep breathing to calm a raging hot flash; practice it regularly to help avoid the onset of hot flashes throughout the day and night. Deep, paced breathing is a strong tool for calming the body and the mind—and it's an incredibly easy technique to use. If you feel a hot flash coming on, begin taking deep, slow breaths through your nose. Breathe in to expand your lungs as far as you can, then hold the breath there for a few seconds before you slowly release it. Let your belly swell out and your chest expand as you breathe in, so your body is fully "inflating" with the breath. When you exhale, empty your lungs completely. Take at least three full, deep breaths and try to remain calm to diminish the hot flash.

A daily program of meditation and relaxation is a powerful tool for keeping your body calm, focused, and strong throughout the day. Its stress-relieving benefits can help ward off hot flashes and other stress-related symptoms of menopause. A ten-minute relaxation session is easy to fit into your morning and evening schedule, and it's easy to do. Sit or lie down in a quiet place with your eyes closed. Consciously relax every muscle in your body, beginning with your feet and continuing the relaxation up toward your head. Concentrate on a single word or object that has personal meaning for you; if other ideas, worries, or mental chatter enter your mind, dismiss them and return to the thought of your focus word. After ten minutes, open your eyes, remain seated, and take three deep breaths before continuing on with your day.

Yoga is an excellent practice for increasing flexibility, building muscle strength and endurance, and eliminating the negative effects of stress on your body. Practicing yoga stretches for twenty to thirty minutes, three times a week can help reduce the negative effects of stress on your body, as it stretches your muscles, improves your balance, and encourages deep, full breathing. Regular yoga practice can also help reduce insomnia, so you fall asleep faster and stay asleep longer. All of these benefits can help eliminate the anxiety triggers that can contribute to hot flashes.

CHAPTER 17

Finding Your New Sexuality

Among the many changes you may experience during perimenopause and menopause is a changing sexual attitude—and appetite. Your age and hormone levels don't determine your sexuality; you are who you have always been, and your fundamental feelings and attitudes about sex don't change when you stop ovulating. But the physical and emotional evolution of a maturing mind and body can color your sexual response.

Checking Your Sexual Attitude

Your attitudes about sex and your own sexuality today are greatly influenced by the attitudes you had about these issues when you were younger. If you enjoyed sex and expected to be sexually satisfied when you were thirty, you're more likely to continue to enjoy sex as you move through your fifties and beyond. Nevertheless, some women report a declining interest in sex after menopause, and most experts agree that changes in attitude accompanied by changes in physical health play a strong role in that shift.

Here are some common reasons women may experience a decline in sexual interest:

- Painful intercourse, resulting from vaginal dryness and atrophy
- Lack of a partner or a partner's declining ability to satisfy
- Feelings of low self-esteem or physical undesirability
- Feeling too tired, too busy, or otherwise preoccupied to enjoy sexual activity

Don't let illness, side effects of medication, or a reluctance to discuss sexual issues with your doctor stand in the way of your ability to enjoy an active sex life. Talk to your doctor or health care provider about changes in your sexual ability or desire. Maintaining your sexual health is important to your overall physical and emotional well-being.

Every woman has unique sexual needs and interests, and many women (and men) have a limited sexual desire at some point in their lives. But if you find your interest in sex waning—at any age—it's important for you to understand why. Maintaining and nurturing your sexuality is important for your physical and emotional health. You shouldn't expect to stop enjoying sex as you age. It's well worth your time to take steps to keep your sex drive alive and thriving through menopause and beyond.

Overcoming Physical Barriers

If you don't feel physically fit and healthy, you're less likely to enjoy an active, healthy sex life. Although you can't postpone menopause or the effects of aging indefinitely, you don't have to let some of the physical symptoms of menopause prevent you from remaining sexually active. If physical problems are interfering with your sexual desire or ability—from vaginal atrophy or incontinence to fatigue resulting from sleep disturbances, illness, or medication—the first step toward resolving those problems is to talk with your gynecologist or other health care provider. Your doctor can recommend treatment options, exercise, dietary or medication changes, or other therapeutic solutions that can lessen or even resolve your physical barriers to an enjoyable sex life. And, as with all aspects of your health care, you may be able to improve your sexual health through some changes in your lifestyle choices.

The Basics

Your daily practices play a big role in your overall fitness—you know that. The same stresses, habits, and substances that damage other aspects of your health can limit your desire and ability to enjoy sex, as well. Here are some basics for maintaining your sexual fitness:

- **Eat right and exercise regularly:** Nutrition and exercise are critical to your overall health as you age, and they play an important role in preserving your sexual health. Regular aerobic, weight-bearing, and stretching exercises keep your body feeling active and alive. Middle age weight gain and ebbing muscle strength and endurance can erode your sexual desire. When your body is strong and fit, you're more energetic and you take a greater interest in all aspects of your life—including sex. If your body is strong and healthy, you're less likely to think of it as an aging relic, and you're more likely to enjoy sharing it with a partner. Plus, exercise releases endorphins, the "feel happy" neurotransmitters in your brain. If you feel better about your body, you're more likely to feel good about sharing it with someone physically. Read Chapters 13, "Eating for a Healthy Menopause," and

14, "Building Exercise into Your Menopause Plan," for diet and exercise ideas.

- **Rest and manage stress:** If your daily routine is too overwhelming to allow you to enjoy an active sex life, it's probably damaging your health in other ways. Stress can lead to headaches, indigestion, muscle pain, depression, and—not surprisingly—a diminished desire for and response to sexual activity. Try to learn what's causing your stress, then do what you can to avoid the stressors. Talk with family and friends, remember to exercise regularly, and learn and practice regular relaxation techniques.

- **Cut down on alcohol and stop smoking:** Most medical experts agree that one or two alcoholic drinks a day aren't bad for your health (unless you have conditions or are taking medication that precludes the use of any alcohol). But drinking too much alcohol can lead to depression, weight gain, and—in some cases—an increased stress response. Smoking fuels stress, as well, and it saps your body of strength and energy. All of these effects can erode your interest in sexual activity and dampen your response to sexual stimulation.

FACTS

Exercise offers a number of benefits for women at any age, but did you know that it could give you a real sexual boost? Some studies have shown that people who practice some form of regular exercise achieve orgasm more easily than do people who don't exercise at all.

- **Treat vaginal dryness:** If you suffer from vaginal dryness or atrophy, intercourse can be painful. Estrogen replacement can help relieve vaginal dryness and keep vaginal tissues moist, elastic, and healthy (see Chapter 11 for more information on the benefits and risks of HRT). Women who cannot use estrogen replacement therapy (such as a woman with a personal history of breast cancer) now have newer options available, such as estrogen suppositories (one brand is Vagifem) that act only in the vagina, which allows for the beneficial effects of estrogen to work where it is needed. Because it is not absorbed into the woman's general circulation, it does not increase the risk of a recurrence of the breast cancer or other estrogen-sensitive conditions.

Improve Sexual Response with the Kegel Exercise

You've probably heard of the Kegel exercise; many women use them to return the strength and condition of their vaginal muscles after childbirth. Other women use the Kegel exercise to improve their ability to control stress incontinence, a problem that many women develop as they approach menopause. Kegel exercise has also been shown to offer women another important benefit: Strengthening vaginal muscles can increase sexual health and pleasure.

The exercises strengthen the pelvic floor muscles that extend from the pubic bone to the tailbone and surround your vaginal opening and the opening to your urinary tract. Strengthening these muscles enables you to contract your vaginal opening, increasing the amount and intensity of the contact between your vagina and your partner's penis. Kegel exercise also increases the blood flow to (and the sensitivity of) your genital area. Practicing them regularly can increase the physical sensations of intercourse, making sex more pleasurable for both you and your partner.

FACTS

Los Angeles obstetrician/gynecologist Arnold Kegel developed the exercise named for him in the mid-1940s as a nonsurgical solution for his patients who were battling incontinence. He later realized that the exercises helped new mothers recover from the physical effects of labor and vaginal childbirth. Today, many women do the Kegel exercise to make their vaginal muscles stronger and more resilient in preparation for childbirth.

You can find your vaginal muscles the next time you urinate. When you begin urinating, squeeze your muscles to stop the flow. Try to start and stop the flow several times, in the same sitting. The muscles you're contracting are those of your pelvic floor musculature—the same set of muscles that you exercise with the Kegel exercise. Once you learn to identify and contract that muscle, you can do your exercises anywhere.

Just contract the pelvic floor muscle and hold it for a count of five. Breathe normally and repeat the contraction, hold, and release ten times. Do this exercise every day—do a dozen repetitions when you're sitting and waiting for a red light to change, or when you're on hold for a phone call. After a month or two of practice, you should notice that you have more control over your bladder and some improved sensation during sexual activity (even masturbation).

Enjoying Your Body

If you lead a hectic life, filled with the responsibilities of work, home, and family, you may have little time to think about yourself—your body, your mind, your pleasure. As your body begins to change with age, it's easy to begin to think of it as your enemy. Something you've always depended on (though you may not have lavished much attention on it) that's letting you down just when you need it most. Many women simply lose touch with their physicality, choosing to ignore their physical condition and respond in the out-of-sight-out-of-mind approach we all know so well.

ESSENTIALS

A multivitamin-mineral supplement may be an easy and inexpensive way to promote your sexuality—and your general health. Vitamin E has been shown in some studies to increase sexual desire, and zinc may help foster sexual arousal (oysters are high in zinc). Selenium is another mineral that is the subject of ongoing studies of sexuality.

The truth is that your body matters; your physical needs matter, too. If you find yourself looking at your body with disappointment or wanting to ignore your body and its physical condition and needs, take conscious action to overcome those feelings. Your body is yours for life, and keeping it healthy, vital, and fit as you approach menopause has never been more important.

All of this book's recommendations for exercise, health care, regular checkups, relaxation techniques, hair and skin treatments, and good diet have been aimed at the important goal of taking care of your body so you can enjoy it. Spending time caring for your body will encourage you to take pleasure in its strength and capabilities. By feeling confident and at ease about your body, you're more likely to enjoy the pleasures of its sexual responses. Learn to include your sexuality in your self-identity; humans are sexual beings, and sexual enjoyment is good for both the body and the mind.

Explore your sexual interests and fantasies. Don't feel ashamed of your sexual orientation, desires, or needs. Many doctors and sex therapists encourage their patients to masturbate to increase their ability to respond to sexual stimulation and to combat stress and anxiety. If you'd like more information on how to become aroused and stay stimulated (by yourself or with a partner), visit your local bookstore, which is full of self-help books on improving your sexual response. Even reading a steamy novel can help you to become aroused. Or rent a film with some love scenes featuring a favorite movie star. You don't have to turn to pornography, just allow yourself to explore and enjoy the sexual arousal you might normally hold back.

Take Your Partner Along for the Ride

If you are in a committed relationship as you near midlife, the chances are good that your partner in that relationship is aging, too. His or her sexual performance and desire may be suffering as much—or even more— than your own. If you and your partner experience a decline in sexual intimacy, you should talk about it.

Many couples ignore sexual problems because they're too embarrassed to discuss them together—let alone with a doctor or other health care professional. But most sexual issues don't resolve themselves. Even if you take action to improve your own sexual response and desire, your partner may not benefit from your experience. In fact, some men and women can feel a bit overwhelmed by their partner's increased sexual desire. So talking with your partner is your first step to getting your sex life back on track.

If your partner is suffering from physical problems that are affecting his or her sexual performance, talking with a doctor is the next step. A general practitioner or gynecologist may decide to refer you to a sex therapist, if your condition warrants that treatment. Keep an open mind and follow your doctor's recommendations. Again, maintaining the health of your sexual relationship is an important part of remaining healthy and happy together.

FACTS

As he ages, your male partner may need more stimulation in order to achieve an erection. As you're learning to enjoy your sexuality more, don't forget to pay attention to your partner's needs. Many couples find that as their sexual relationship matures they draw increasing pleasure from the nonintercourse parts of their lovemaking, and use their hands and mouths more frequently during sex.

Enhancing Your Sexual Experience

You may find that your lovemaking simply needs some new life. Take this opportunity to enjoy a second "first romance" with your partner. Learn to touch each other again and take pleasure in your physical contact; take baths and showers together and spend more time in touching and foreplay during lovemaking. Let your partner know what feels good to you and find out what he or she enjoys most, and explore your fantasies. Don't forget to use vaginal creams and lubricants to make the sexual experience more enjoyable. (If you're using condoms, remember to use water-based lubricants; petroleum can weaken the condom wall and cause breaks and tears.) At this stage in your life, you can move beyond the shyness and embarrassment of adolescence. Your bodies are yours to enjoy, so don't hold back.

Be Creative

Don't become complacent about your sex life. Many women expect spontaneous bursts of admiration from their partners, even if they haven't been demonstrating much interest in their body or their sexuality lately. If you've stopped paying attention to your physical appearance, take some time to do the things that will make you look and feel more beautiful. Get a new haircut or have a facial. Stop by the cosmetics counter at your local department store, and ask for some ideas for revitalizing your appearance. When you look better, you feel more sexually appealing.

It you're having sex with multiple partners, don't forget to be scrupulously clean and use condoms for protection from sexually transmitted diseases. And if you haven't gone at least twelve months without a period (or were diagnosed as menopausal through a blood test), you can still be fertile, so use appropriate birth control measures.

Would a new nightgown or dressing gown make you feel sexier? Silky, flattering lingerie comes in a variety of styles and sizes, so visit a lingerie store to check out your options. If you've grown self-conscious about your midlife physique, wearing a flattering negligee during lovemaking can help you feel more confident and relaxed. And while you're there, try some of the new bust-shaping brassieres. Many women in midlife have a cleavage for the first time, so why not take advantage of it?

Setting the mood is all-important for revitalizing your lovemaking. Lower the lights, burn some aromatic candles, and play some soft, sensual music. Now is the time to relax and explore sensual pleasures. Put away the sweatpants and dress for dinner—if you're dining at home, why not try a "French maid" costume? Use your imagination and have fun with sex. Be creative, experiment, and try to be open with your partner about your feelings and responses to whatever you experience together.

CHAPTER 18

Overcoming Mood Swings, Anxiety, and Depression

Many women do experience depression, anxiety, and/or mood swings during perimenopause. Mood disorders can be triggered by a number of causes, and if you suffer from them—at any time during your life—it's important that you understand the source of your problems as well as how best to treat them. Through medical treatment, stress management, and smart lifestyle choices, you can learn to regain control of your emotional stability.

Looking Stress in the Eye

Stress is a fact of life for everyone, and women approaching the age of menopause certainly aren't immune from its effects. In fact, women in perimenopause may be more susceptible to the health-damaging side effects of stress than they have been at previous times in their lives. Stress exacerbates a wide range of medical problems, from stomach disorders and headaches to insomnia and even depression. Stress can be a major contributor to mood swings, anxiety, and mild depression, so if you suffer from these emotional disorders, one of your first steps toward recovery may be to identify the sources of stress in your life.

Women in midlife can be faced with any number of stressors, including career and financial issues, body image changes, emerging health problems, divorce, widowhood, struggles with teenage children, and increasing responsibilities for aging parents. Though many women will have dealt with some or all of these issues at previous times in life, the added stress of adjusting to hormonal fluctuations, hot flashes, weight gain, or other potential side effects of perimenopause can make the burden of stress even harder to bear during midlife.

ESSENTIALS   Learn to delegate responsibilities; if you do this early, before the pressure really builds up, you're less likely to crack.

Some of the most common symptoms of stress include headaches, sleeplessness, indigestion, forgetfulness, an inability to concentrate, and ongoing feelings of anger and unhappiness. Stress can leave you feeling drained of all good feeling, and it can lead to overeating, drinking too much alcohol, or stepping up the pace of other unhealthy stress habits such as cigarette smoking. If you experience any of these symptoms of stress, you need to realize that you have a real, health-threatening problem and take action to determine its sources and potential solutions. Unless you find ways to eliminate or manage stress, you won't be successful in combating the mood-related problems you may experience during perimenopause.

Managing Stress

You can't avoid all sources of stress, but you may be able to find workarounds for many of them. For example, if a hectic work and family schedule is depleting your energy and contributing to stress, try to see what activities you can trim from your list of daily activities. Can you ask a partner for help in managing household tasks or running errands? Can you afford to hire a service to do laundry, pick up and deliver dry cleaning, or take over major cleaning jobs around the house? If you have children, can you ask them to step up to the plate and take more responsibility for their own needs or to help out more around the house? If aging parents are presenting increasing demands on your time, can you get any type of community support assistance, such as meal deliveries, or the services of a visiting nurse?

And don't stop at examining your home and family responsibilities, either. Evaluate your job and work habits to try to spot stress fixes there, as well. Can you ask your boss for flexible work times, so you can schedule your commute when traffic is less hectic, or even arrange to work at home one day a week? Can you find someone to carpool with? If you commute by train, can you do some of your work on a laptop computer, and save time at the office? If you have problems with a co-worker, can you schedule a meeting to try to resolve the issues, or at least to lessen the tension? Can a personal organizer, meeting scheduler program, or other software help you save time and cut down on unnecessary panic and last-minute emergencies? Can you ask a well-organized coworker for help in finding ways to trim the fat from your work habits?

FACTS

Don't assume that you absolutely *must* or *can't* do anything. This isn't a time to mindlessly adhere to old routines or to be driven by false necessity; rethink your priorities and learn to devote your time and attention to the things that serve you best.

When you've pinpointed and reduced the stressors that you can, find ways to cope with the stress you can't get rid of. Exercise regularly, spend time engaged in leisure activities you enjoy, eat a healthy diet, and go easy on your mind and body—don't expect to perform every task flawlessly and on time.

Whatever the possible solutions, the first key to relieving stress is to come to grips with the fact that stress presents a real health risk—one you simply cannot overlook. Stress will wear you out, age your body and mind, drain your spirit, and cause serious and lasting health problems. Though you may feel that you have no options—that you're stuck with the stressful situations you currently endure—you do have options available to you. Talk to your doctor, a therapist, a counselor, a friend, a minister, or a trusted family member, and ask for help in finding ways to manage stress.

Your stress may be connected to a medical condition or the medication or treatment program you're using to combat one. Your doctor or health care provider may be able to adjust your medication or offer additional treatment options that can help you reduce and manage any health-related stressors you're encountering.

Recognize the Symptoms

Nearly 25 percent of all women suffer from some form of depression at some time during their lives. Many studies have shown that women first experience depression when they're in their twenties, or even younger. And although menopause doesn't automatically signal the onset of depression, women who have suffered from depression earlier in life, or women who have had postpartum depression or even severe premenstrual syndrome (PMS), are more likely to have recurring depression during perimenopause. Women who have a family history of depression also run more risk of suffering from depression during perimenopause.

Many researchers believe that the physical changes of perimenopause—the fluctuating levels of estrogen and progesterone many women experience during this time—can contribute to mood swings and other emotional symptoms of perimenopause, though the mechanisms of their impact are under continual study. Doctors know, however, that estrogen is directly related to our body's production of serotonin—an important chemical that works in the brain to regulate moods. As estrogen levels shift, so does the brain's supply of serotonin—and therefore, moods can shift, as well.

But body chemistry isn't the only thing that can trigger midlife mood decay. Women who are dealing with changing roles at home or at work, changing levels of energy, or diminishing feelings of general fitness and well-being are at risk of suffering from emotional upheavals and imbalances.

ESSENTIALS

As you move into perimenopause, it's important that you remain aware of your feelings and alert for signs of emotional problems. Just as you have to check up on and monitor your physical health regularly, you need to watch for and deal with symptoms of emotional disorder to maintain your overall fitness and well-being.

Coming to grips with your emotional upsets by recognizing symptoms and tracking them to their source can be a first step toward resolving the problem. When you have some understanding of the types and severity of the symptoms you're experiencing, you're better able to determine your next course of action. You may be able to control mild mood disturbances simply by changing your diet, exercise program, or reactions to certain stress-inducing stimuli. Such techniques are covered later in this chapter along with information about medication, counseling, and other treatment options that can help restore your emotional order and balance when lifestyle and behavioral changes aren't enough.

Tracking Your Mood Swings

Mood shifts are relatively mild changes in mood that can quickly take a woman from feelings of joy, to anger, fatigue, or despair. The triggers for these responses can be unpredictable—and sometimes, seemingly inconsequential. Perimenopausal women who report mood swings cite a wide range of stimuli for these events. If you're swinging, you can be moved to tears by a song on the radio or the color of the light as evening falls over your backyard. You can become incredibly angry when a coworker asks for clarification of a point you made in a memo, when children or a partner fail to take care of their household responsibilities, or when you forget to stop and pick up the dry cleaning on your way home. Mood swings can sometimes be no more than a normal response, magnified to a level much higher than normal.

ESSENTIALS

During perimenopause, mood swings simply indicate that your body and mind are adjusting to a variety of physical, emotional, and social changes that accompany this phase of your life. Though it's easy to dismiss these emotions as being "just the change," don't fail to recognize them as your response to some real experience or stimulus.

You may be reacting to some source of irritation, unhappiness, discomfort, fear, love, joy, or longing. As estrogen levels rise and fall due to your body's release of the hormone, serotonin levels can rise and fall, too, taking your mood right along with them. Or, mood swings can be a response to a medical condition or chemical imbalance in your body— one, perhaps, that can be treated through counseling, medication, or other therapy. Your mood swings can teach you a lot about who you are, what issues and changes you're dealing with, and where you want to go during this transition in your life.

You can expect some mood swings in your life, especially as you reach midlife. But many women in perimenopause develop mood swings that interfere with their lives. Frequent or severe mood swings can create problems with family, coworkers, and friends; cause missed workdays; discourage participation in social functions or enjoyable activities; or create feelings of alienation, exhaustion, fear, and a lack of control. If mood swings are severe or frequent enough to get in the way of your full—and fulfilling—life, take action to bring them under control.

The Symptoms of Anxiety

Anxiety is a natural, healthy response to certain realities of life— beginning a new job, meeting upcoming deadlines, passing examinations, and so on. But anxiety that interferes with your ability to function at full capacity throughout your day and then sleep soundly throughout the night is definitely unhealthy. Anxiety can be a side effect of a more serious mood-destabilizing condition—depression.

Anxiety can be associated with depression, or it can be a side effect of sleeplessness, excess fatigue, or unmanageable levels of stress. Many people suffering from anxiety describe it as overwhelming feelings of fear, nervousness, or the conviction that something dreadful is about to happen—though they often can't pinpoint what that something may be. When these feelings begin to interfere with normal, everyday functioning, they may represent an anxiety disorder. Some other symptoms of anxiety include:

- An unshakable feeling of fear, dread, or worry that lasts for more than three days
- Chest pain, racing heart, or fast breathing
- Stomach pain, cramps, or diarrhea
- Hand-wringing, pacing, or other repetitive nervous movement

FACTS

Women in perimenopause sometimes report the occurrence of panic attacks—overwhelming feelings of intense fear or impending doom that occur suddenly and repeatedly. Symptoms include shortness of breath, choking sensations, heart pounding or palpitations, and the sensation of losing control.

Anxiety that goes unchecked can develop into anxiety disorders. These disorders include social phobias, such as agoraphobia (fear of going out in public), specific phobias (such as fear of dogs or spiders), or obsessive behaviors (such as obsessive hand washing or repeatedly checking door locks or appliance switches).

Know the Symptoms of Depression

Though transient feelings of sadness, despair, or a general dissatisfaction with life are common during perimenopause, if these feelings are long-lasting or severe, they could be signaling the onset of depression. Insomnia, fatigue, hot flashes, and other perimenopausal symptoms can trigger minor mood disorders during perimenopause. But major depression goes well beyond the typical reaction to these perimenopausal symptoms. Though sometimes doctors can't identify the cause, major depression is often the result of a biological or chemical imbalance that requires careful diagnosis and treatment.

According to the North American Menopause Society, women are more likely than men to increase their consumption of alcohol when depressed. Abusing alcohol or drugs compounds the problems of midlife, and women in perimenopause should be wary of self-medicating with these substances.

Sometimes, depression itself can be a symptom or side effect of some major life event, such as a divorce, the death of a loved one, losing a job, or dealing with a severe or ongoing medical problem—all problems that can occur to women at midlife. But these sorts of event-triggered depressions may pass with time or resolve themselves quickly, without the need for special treatment or therapy. Sometimes, however, these events can lead to depression that deepens into a more systemic, major depression that women are unlikely to overcome without some form of treatment.

The characteristic symptoms of major depression follow:

- Feelings of hopelessness, worthlessness, guilt, or a general depressed mood that lasts most of the day, nearly every day for two weeks or longer
- Fatigue and loss of energy
- Difficulty concentrating
- Loss of interest in activities you previously found to be pleasurable
- Sleep disorder, whether sleeping too much or suffering from insomnia
- Recurrent thoughts of suicide or death

Major depression is an illness, with many options for treatment. If you suffer from depression, the sooner you get help, the more quickly and effectively you can overcome the physical and emotional side effects of this devastating condition.

FACTS

Depression can harm you, your family, your job, and your friends and coworkers. Those around you are likely to be confused, saddened, worried, or even irritated by your depressed behavior. Don't let your depression become "contagious"; talk to a health professional or trusted advisor to get the help you need.

Take Action

You may have difficulty recognizing that you are suffering from an emotional imbalance or mood disorder. Many women can go through months of emotional turmoil thinking, "It's just a bad day," then "What a bad week," to "This month has been awful," and still believe that they're just feeling temporarily down, moody, or out of sorts. Often, these women are taken aback when a friend, spouse, or relative expresses concerns over their moodiness, irritability, or remoteness.

If you or those around you suspect that your emotional behavior may signal a mood disorder, you need to take action to seek a diagnosis and, if necessary, make behavioral changes or begin treatment. Your goal is to get your life back in balance, so you can regain your sense of confidence and purpose.

Rule Out Medical Causes

Mood swings, depression, and anxiety can be triggered or made worse by medical problems. Thyroid disorders can sometimes result in depression, as can the use of some medications used to treat hypertension. Some weight-loss drugs can trigger a rise in anxiety levels or even panic attacks. As you seek to find the causes and solutions for your emotional imbalances, begin by talking with your gynecologist or general practitioner. That individual can review your medications and health history to uncover any potential medical causes for your mood disorders.

Your doctor or health care provider can also uncover contributing medical conditions, such as insomnia, sleep apnea, or extreme hormonal imbalances, that may contribute to your mood swings. If your doctor uncovers specific medical causes for your condition, he or she can adjust your medication, treat the contributing medical condition, or suggest other specific treatment options best suited to resolving those issues.

Explore Your Treatment Options

When medical complications have been ruled out, you have several treatment options available to you for diminishing—or even eliminating—your mood disorder symptoms. The option that's best for you is determined, in part, by the severity of your problem and your personal and family medical history.

Stress can trigger the biological changes that accompany depression, and it appears that hormonal shifts can trigger those changes, too. That's why women with a family or personal history of depression must be particularly careful to monitor and manage stress as they approach the age of menopause.

If you suffer from major depression, your doctor is likely to prescribe some sort of antidepressant medication. (See the section For Combating Insomnia, Depression, and Anxiety in Chapter 12.) Following is a quick list of some of the most commonly prescribed antidepressant and antianxiety medications:

- Selective serotonin reuptake inhibitors (SSRIs), including fluoxetine, sertraline, and paroxetine (marketed as Prozac, Zoloft, and Paxil). Though SSRIs can cause depressed sexual response and other side effects in certain individuals, they are nonaddictive and work by helping your body make better use of the serotonin it naturally produces. Fluoxetine is also approved for premenstrual dysphoric disorder (PMDD) and is available as a once-a-week timed-release dosage.

- Antianxiety drugs, or anxiolytics—such as buspirone and alprazolam—can lessen the effects of depression, anxiety, and sleeplessness, and they also can treat the symptoms of PMDD that many perimenopausal women experience as they move closer to menopause. Anxiolytics can have a slightly sedative effect, so many doctors prescribe them for short periods of time only.

ESSENTIALS

Many doctors prescribe antidepressants in combination with hormone replacement therapy for perimenopausal or menopausal women with severe depression. Though HRT is rarely the first-course treatment for depression, it can alleviate symptoms such as hot flashes and insomnia that contribute to depression, and it offers other benefits for menopausal women. (See Chapter 11 for more information.)

Psychological counseling—psychotherapy—is a powerful treatment option for women experiencing excess anxiety, stress, or mood disturbance during perimenopause and menopause. Most studies have shown that counseling in conjunction with antidepressant medication offers more long-term and effective results than does a treatment using medication alone. Though you may not experience the benefits of psychotherapy immediately after you begin treatment, its effects can be long-lasting and wide-reaching.

The two types of psychotherapy you are most likely to receive for emotional problems associated with perimenopause are interpersonal therapy or cognitive-behavioral therapy. Interpersonal therapy explores the relationships in your life and how they may be contributing to your emotional problems. This type of therapy also teaches you how you may use the strength and support you gain from your relationships to help deal with emotional issues. Cognitive-behavioral therapy examines your core thoughts and beliefs and how they determine your actions in response to life. If you have developed a pessimistic or negative attitude toward life in general, this type of therapy can help you see the world in a more balanced perspective and learn more effective ways of viewing and coping with life.

FACTS

Learning to be optimistic can have real physical and emotional health benefits. Though no conclusive studies have proven the benefits of optimism, many medical professionals have observed that their pessimistic patients are prone to have an elevated blood pressure, less resistance to disease, and a slower recovery time following illnesses or injury.

Staying "On the Level"

If you are experiencing mild mood disturbances, anxiety, or general but recurring feelings of the blues, you have a number of simple self-treatment options for leveling out the emotional roller-coaster ride.

First, give your body and mind healthy amounts of good fuel, activity, and rest. Eat a healthy diet that emphasizes fruit, vegetables, and whole grains and skips high-fat, low-nutrient foods loaded with sugar, salt, and simple carbohydrates. Limiting the amount of caffeine, salt, MSG, and sugar you consume can help your body remain active and alert, rather than jumpy and fatigued. Your physical and emotional health are inextricably linked, and you can't maintain either with a crummy diet.

Here are some other good guidelines to follow:

- **Eat sensible amounts of food throughout the day.** If you stuff yourself or try to eat your way out of a low mood, you just add to the problem by contributing to weight gain, low self-esteem, and poor body image. But if you skip meals or rely on junk food or fast-food fixes because you're just too busy to worry about when and what you're eating, you can stress both your body and mind—and rob them of the nutrients they need. If a lack of time is a problem, check out the frozen foods section of your grocery. Lots of frozen meals are tasty, nutritious, and low in fat and calories. Bad nutrition can lead to illness, fatigue, and a host of other problems that can leave you feeling hopeless and depressed. Caring about your body is essential to caring for your mind.

- **Be active.** Though mood swings, anxiety, and depression can leave you feeling frozen—uninterested in life and incapable of doing anything to participate in it—activity is one of the best ways to lift and stabilize your mood. Physical activity triggers your body to releases mood-lifting endorphins, and it gets your heart pumping to circulate healthy, oxygenated blood throughout your body. Participating in activities with family and friends can help lighten your mood, broaden your perspective on the issues that are troubling you, and renew your hopes and interests so you can deal more effectively with issues that threaten your emotional health. Get involved in activities that challenge both mind and body, pick up a hobby, or revisit old interests that engage your creativity and motivate you to exercise your talents. Physical activity and regular exercise actually leave you feeling more energetic.

- **Practice meditation or relaxation techniques.** Meditation, relaxation techniques, and mind-body exercises such as yoga and t'ai chi are powerful tools for relieving hot flashes and other symptoms of stress, anxiety, and mild depression. (See the section on Mind-Body Exercises in Chapter 16 for more information on these techniques.) Fifteen-minute sessions of meditation, deep breathing, or relaxation every morning and evening can help reduce or even eliminate much of the stress and mood-altering emotional upheavals of perimenopause.

- **Get plenty of rest.** Try to establish and maintain a regular sleep schedule, in which you go to sleep and rise at the same times every day—including weekends. Take time to read, listen to music, or soak in a hot tub to relax and prepare yourself for sleep. Don't exercise or eat large amounts of food late in the evening.

ALERT

If you find yourself awakening and unable to return to sleep early in the morning for more than three or four days in a row, you should contact your doctor or health care professional. Re-establishing a healthy sleep pattern is essential to maintaining good health; the longer your sleep is disturbed, the more difficulty you'll have returning to a normal cycle.

You Don't Have to Go It Alone

No one treatment option is right—or even effective—for every woman. But any woman suffering from mood disorders should talk with a doctor, counselor, mentor, or other trusted advisor to discuss all appropriate treatments. Depression and other mood disturbances are not a typical byproduct of the aging process. A willingness to admit and discuss mood disorders is your best weapon for overcoming them.

Though women are statistically more likely than men to suffer from depression, they are also more likely to look for help in overcoming issues that affect their emotional health. Your friends, family, coworkers, doctors, minister, or other counselors can help you find ways to put emotional issues to rest, so you can concentrate on becoming healthier, stronger, and more engaged in life as each year passes.

CHAPTER 19

Keeping
Your Mind Sharp

With our bodies living longer than at any time in history, our surest chance for a happy and independent old age lies in keeping our minds as finely tuned and functional as possible—for as long as we possibly can.

How Your Brain Changes as You Age

Most medical and scientific authorities agree that the mind's ability to think clearly and quickly changes with age, but those changes aren't linked to menopause. The brain doesn't have a "use by" shelf life exactly; most nerves are capable of lasting one hundred years or more. But changes in the brain's physical size and functions do occur with age, and those changes can have an impact on how well you can recall information stored in your brain.

The human brain shrinks slightly after age fifty as a result of a loss of water content. The shrinkage itself doesn't impair your memory, but the loss of frontal-lobe volume that accompanies that loss can. Some neuroscientists believe frontal lobes can shrink up to 30 percent between the ages of fifty and ninety. Frontal lobes are critical to complex thinking—your ability to reason, pay attention, and perform multiple tasks at the same time. A diminished capacity in your frontal lobes can diminish your abilities in all of these cognitive functions.

FACTS

If you plan to live for a long time, you need to take good care of your mind. Want to calculate how long you're likely to live? Go to *www.beeson.org/livingto100/* to take Dr. Thomas Perls's Living to 100 Life Expectancy Calculator, presented by the Alliance for Aging Research.

Perhaps most important to preserving memory and recall is the brain's hippocampus—the part of the brain where memory is stored, created, and retrieved. Some researchers believe the hippocampus can lose ability with age—resulting in a slowdown of the brain's ability to store and retrieve memory. Exacerbating this slowdown are metabolic changes and a dwindling number of dendrites—the neurons that transmit the brain's signals. All of these changes can combine to make your brain feel duller and slower.

You don't need to panic that you're suffering an onset of early Alzheimer's disease every time you misplace your car keys—especially not as you approach the age of menopause. Many of the symptoms of menopause, including mood swings, sleeplessness, increased susceptibility to stress, and fluctuating levels of hormones, can contribute to less efficient cognitive functions—but most of these symptoms are relatively mild and transient.

Take Steps to Keep Your Mind Sharp

You have a number of options available to you for keeping your brain functioning as strongly as possible into and through menopause. But, maintaining good cognitive functions takes effort. You can't just pop a pill or wear a special bracelet to protect your brain's functions. The first step toward maintaining a healthy, active brain is to maintain a healthy, active body. That requires good nutrition (including proper nutritional supplements) and regular exercise.

Most experts agree that all individuals age fifty and over are wise to take steps to preserve their cognitive strength. Even at advanced ages the mind continues to be capable of learning and recalling new information—but that type of mental fitness requires effort.

Give Your Brain the Nutrition It Needs

Your brain needs fuel in order to function. Some experts estimate that the brain uses 20 percent or more of the body's energy. Glucose and antioxidants are important components of your brain's nutrition, so make sure your diet includes plenty of whole grains, fruit, and vegetables. The brain also may benefit from folates—found in leafy green vegetables, lentils, and other legumes. Folic acid, a laboratory produced version of folate, is included in many multivitamins and some fortified foods. Many studies also show that daily recommended doses of vitamin E and selenium may help slow the diminishment of cognitive functions. Recently, Lipoic acid and Coenzyme Q have been recognized to improve brain health, cognitive function, and memory.

Doctors have found that estrogen helps aid the brain's functions of remembering and storing new information, so estrogen therapy can help postpone a decline in cognitive functions and protect short-term and long-term memory. Estrogen also helps improve the circulation to the brain by directly dilating the critical blood vessels involved. If you are taking estrogen therapy or HRT as part of your general menopausal health maintenance plan, you can add this benefit to the many others you'll receive from that therapy.

Exercise Your Body to Keep Your Brain Healthy

Regular exercise—at least twenty minutes a day, but thirty minutes to an hour daily is best—is one great way to preserve your mental acuity. Aerobic exercise helps get the blood coursing through your system, carrying oxygen and glucose to your brain—two substances the brain needs in order to function.

Regular exercise also can prod the brain into producing more molecules that help protect and produce the brain's neurons. Though studies are still underway to establish the link between exercise and increased brain neurons, many researchers—including those involved with Alzheimer's disease research—are studying the protective effects of regular physical exercise on the brain's neural paths for transmitting signals.

FACTS

Physical exercise is a great way to reduce stress, and stress can take a serious toll on cognitive functions. Stress inhibits your ability to concentrate and it can shorten your lifespan. The New England Centenarian Study has found that one trait common among those who live beyond the age of one hundred is an ability to handle stress. (See Chapter 18 for other recommended stress-busters.)

Exercise Your Brain to Keep It Lively

Some simple, but effective, techniques for putting your mind through some hoops to keep it active and highly functional are presented later in this chapter. But many of the most important things you can do to hone your memory are really just good habits—things you do every day as a matter of course that keep your brain's neurons charged and firing, and your hippocampus fully loaded and ready to dispense information.

Mental exercise can increase the size of different areas of the brain, just as physical exercise increases muscle size. Researchers have long known that musicians' brains are different in proportion than those of non-musicians, but a study of the brains of London cab drivers, reported in March 2000, indicated that this effect can continue into late adulthood. London cabbies are required to spend two years memorizing all of the streets, back alleys, shops, and businesses in London—information known as "the Knowledge"—then pass a memory test to get their licenses. Researchers found that the brain of a trained and licensed cabbie had a hippocampus larger than that area in the brains of a control group. And the hippocampus continued to enlarge as the cabbie used the Knowledge. Cabbies who had been driving for some time—some for over forty years—had a larger hippocampus than their less-experienced colleagues.

SSENTIALS When you're trying to memorize or recall something important, eliminate all other distractions. Turn off the television, lower the volume on the stereo, and get to a quiet place where people aren't chattering around you. You'll find you have to put in less time and effort if you are able to concentrate better, and you'll retain the information longer.

You don't have to build a street map of London in your brain to improve your memory. But you do have to make some effort to "pump up" your memory. Here are some basic brain-building practices:

Pay attention: The first clue to preserving—or even improving—your memory is to learn to pay attention to what is being said and what is happening around you. Many researchers believe that inattentiveness is a major cause of forgetfulness in people of any age. If you don't learn to really listen and observe, your brain has no opportunity to absorb and store information. And pay attention to your actions as well; the classic lost-keys problem is easily resolved by creating a home-base spot where you always put your keys, for example. Write out lists of important things you must do, and read the list out loud as you think about each item and visualize some image or action that each represents to you.

Slow down and repeat information: When you hear a new name or have to commit a list of things to memory, stop, slow down, and repeat the information you have to remember several times. Repeat the name to yourself (other word-association ideas for remembering names appear in the following text), and—if you've just met someone—repeat that person's name during the conversation, as in, "Well, Joanne, have you been living in the area long?" Or "Steve Sampler, that name sounds familiar—do you have relatives living in this area?"

Write it down: Keep a notepad and pen in handy places around the house, for example, next to every telephone, by the front door, and in your car, so you can write down spur-of-the-moment ideas when they occur to you.

Keep thinking: Every day participate in some mental activity that requires your brain to remember, reason, and react quickly. Work a crossword puzzle, play a word game, play chess, put away the calculator and do your own multiplication and division, read a book, debate politics with your partner, draw, paint, play a musical instrument, take a class at the local university or adult learning center, or write in a journal. Vegetating in front of the television may offer a good thirty-minute break from a hectic day, but that shouldn't be your main form of recreation. The more you exercise your brain's ability to think, the better it will function.

Watch out for alcohol and other mind-numbing drugs. Most experts agree that a drink a day isn't health threatening, but drinking too much can deaden your brain's ability to retain and recall information. Abuse of alcohol or recreational drugs can diminish your ability to absorb stimuli from the world around you, and result in a limited ability to form new memories.

Most doctors agree that keeping your memory alive and well is simply a matter of following the basic advice offered throughout this section of the chapter: eat right, exercise your body, and exercise your mind. But, you can use a few memory enhancing quizzes, games, and techniques to build your total recall.

Enhance Your Memory with These Methods

Though most doctors agree that you don't need any formal mental gymnastics to keep your brain fit and functioning, many people have found that certain techniques or activities have helped them hone their memory. The simple techniques offered here can give you a leg up in bolstering your ability to learn and recall new information.

Imagine this scenario: You're getting ready for work in the morning, and one of those morning news television programs is chattering away in the background. You hear one of the announcers mention a product development that gives you an idea for one of the projects your team is involved in at work. You tell yourself you're going to research the product further once you hit the office, and discuss your ideas with your team. But by the time you're backing your car out of the driveway, you've put the whole thing out of your mind. When you get to work, you have a sense that there's something you were going to do, but . . .

Events, ideas, information that pass into the hippocampus will pass right on out again, unless you do something to lock them down—by associating them with other memory that is already safely stored and ready for retrieval. The more associations the memory is tied to, the more likely you are to be able to store and retrieve it later. In psychol-ogy, this technique of associating new information with a range of memories for stronger recall is called elaborative encoding. It takes place in your frontal lobes—an area of your brain that always can use a good workout. Over time, people have used a number of memory devices to aid this process:

Create mental pictographs or visualizations: You've heard the trick of memorizing names by associating each with familiar images—a blue jay reading *Ms.* magazine to a hairless guy with a winning lottery ticket may represent James Baldwin to you, for example. To remember six items you must pick up at the store on the way home, you may create a mental image of a chicken swimming in a kidney-shaped pool full of tomato juice that has a diving board made of a broad stalk of celery. On the edge of the pool rest brown life preservers studded with raisins and a lidded jar of thick sunblock cream. You stop to pick up chicken, kidney beans, tomato juice, celery, raisin bagels, and butter.

Use the "Roman Room": Ancient Romans used this practice to help them memorize long speeches, lists of objects, city names, and so on. To try it, envision a room. Then place around the room visual cues that remind you of items from your to-do list, shopping list, or other types of information. A coat draped over a chair reminds you of the dry cleaning that needs to be picked up. A pair of skis leaning in the corner reminds you to call the travel agent about your plane tickets for your trip to Vermont. Travel around the room in your mind, and make a mental note of sensory cues given off by the items—the colors, sounds, and smells of the items, how they coexist with each other in the room, and any reaction they evoke in you. Make the images as vivid and compelling as possible. The room should continue to exist in your mind as a real place, with each of its furnishings a reminder of the things, people, or events you want to lock in your memory.

Go into training for long-term lockdown: When you have stored information in your long-term memory—not just until you leave work or get through tomorrow's meeting—put your memory technique into a training program. Review the information you need to remember at least three times a day for the next three to five days. At the end of your training program, you should have the information safely in the vault.

Most of all, remember to work hard at preserving and building your cognitive functions, but try to enjoy the ride. After all, if you're worried about your memory, you probably aren't too far down the forgetfulness trail to get your ability to store and recall new information back up to speed.

CHAPTER 20

Keeping a Menopause Journal

A menopause journal can be an important tool for both you and your doctor. By chronicling your experiences, you create a clear vision of the physical and emotional changes you've experienced, to help you understand where you've been—and perhaps, where you're going—as you move into the final third of your life.

Why Should You Keep a Journal?

Perimenopause marks the beginning of another important phase of your life. And keeping a record of your evolution and the milestones you pass along the way can have important benefits for both your body and mind.

FACTS

Writing is good therapy, even for chronic illnesses. In an abstract published in 1999 in the *Journal of the American Medical Association*, doctors reported that writing about the experience of suffering from asthma and arthritis had a "surprisingly beneficial effect on symptom reports, well-being, and health care" for the individuals recording their experiences.

Your Journal as a Medical Record

A menopause journal serves a more serious purpose, but in much the same way. You keep a menopause journal to record the physical and emotional symptoms you experience each day as you move toward and through menopause. Part of your journal will be a medical record, where you list physical observations, such as migraine headaches, irregular periods, sleepless nights, changes in your weight, and so on. This same calendar should include your menstrual periods, so that if an association exists, you or your doctor will be able to notice. You aren't just keeping a record of your symptoms, but their severity, frequency, and recurrence—so you can spot any patterns that occur.

Your doctors will benefit greatly from the information you've recorded in your menopause journal. They can use the information to gain a fuller picture of the way your symptoms are evolving and to gauge your response to medications and other treatment options you're exploring. If certain symptoms occur in tandem or in a specific sequence each month, especially in conjunction with your periods, or with a lack of menstrual bleeding, that information may help your doctors better understand the specific triggering mechanism that prompts them.

Your Journal as a Personal Record

You also can use your journal to record your emotional symptoms and responses to the process of passing through perimenopause and menopause. The very act of writing down your thoughts and feelings is a powerful tool for understanding them. Your journal gives you a much closer look at who you are, who you're becoming, what you most fear, and what your hopes for the future entail. And, the accurate record of the progress and patterns of your symptoms over the months in your journal actually can help you manage your reactions to some menopausal symptoms and expand your understanding of the process you're experiencing.

For example, your journal may record anxiety attacks, and over time, you realize that those that wake you up at three A.M. and cost you hours of sleepless worry occur most often between the tenth through fourteenth days of your cycle. This understanding may enable you to say to yourself, "This panic I'm feeling is a chemical response to hormonal fluctuations, not a true reaction to impending disaster." With that, you may be able to do your deep breathing exercises, calm your mind, and return to sleep more quickly.

ESSENTIALS

Continue your journal after the doctor prescribes any medical or hormonal therapy, or if you add an over-the-counter supplement to your regimen, so that you can gauge any positive result or side effects over time.

If you suffer from stress, simply writing in your journal may give you a means for lessening the effects of this health-eroding condition. By writing about your stress—events that triggered the stress, your reactions, and your thoughts about resolving the stress-inducing issues in your life—you give yourself a moment to stop the cycle of nervous tension, worry, anger, and fear that add fuel and momentum to your stress.

Many women have noted that perimenopause and menopause trigger feelings of introspection they haven't experienced before. If you find yourself thinking about your past, recollecting family vacations, relatives you haven't seen for years, or your old boyfriends, write it down! These thoughts and ideas are important to you right now, or they wouldn't be occupying your mind. Making a record of them helps you take a broader look at exactly what about these past events may be saying to you now. Just remember to keep separate medical and personal journals, or transfer information from one journal into the symptom diary or calendar that you plan to take with you to your doctor's appointments.

FACTS

Interested in seeing what other women write about their experience with menopause? The Discovery Channel hosts one woman's menopause journal online, at ✍ *www.health.discovery.com*. (Go to Women's Health and search under "menopause journal."

Deciding What You Want Your Journal to Be

You can keep your menopause journal in any of a number of different forms and formats. Your journal can be as formal or informal as you choose it to be—you may write in a small, spiral-bound notebook; an unlined composition book; or one of the many leather or clothbound book-length journals for sale in most bookstores today. If you're a dedicated computer user, you may prefer to use any of the many journal-writing software programs, or you may prefer to write in a simple word-processing program and create your own journal organization. Your choices will be determined by when—and how—you use your menopause journal.

If you walk into a large bookstore today, chances are that you'll find a large selection of blank journals, beautifully bound and just waiting for your thoughts. Though you want to make sure that you'll enjoy keeping your journal (so you'll be more inclined to write in it on a regular basis), don't choose a journal format based on its cover appeal. You need a journal that will fit your lifestyle, your writing style, and your habits.

That leather-bound, vellum-leafed book-style journal may make you feel like Jane Austen when you hold it in your hand, but how easy is it to write in? Will it lay open on the desk? Is it easy to balance on your knees? Are the pages too narrow to accommodate more than three words in your open, freehand scrawl? That journaling software may do everything but write your entries for you, but do you find that you're most inspired to write in your journal when you're away from your computer? Are the program's features too difficult to use or in the way for the type of writing you prefer to do?

Your menopause journal will be a very personal document, so only you can decide what shape and form it should be. Are you most comfortable writing by hand or with a keyboard? If you plan to use a computer, you need to be sure that yours is located in an area where you're comfortable relaxing and writing. If your computer is shared with other members of the family, you may prefer to set up some sort of password protection so that you can write what you choose to write, without worrying about family members' reactions.

Taking a hard-copy journal on the road always leaves open the possibility that it will be lost or stolen. Travelers may want to keep a separate road journal and transfer the information to a main journal when they return home. Always make backup copies of electronic journals to prevent a loss due to hard disc failure or other computer-related mishaps.

Journal-writing software, such as LifeJournal, can help your organize, sort, and search your entries to track recurrent physical and emotional issues over time. If you plan to keep a hand-written journal, you'll want to find one that's the right size and shape for the types of records you want to keep. You may not want a week-at-a-glance-type layout, for example, if you want to do free writing, in which you may need ample space to write about your day. If you plan to keep numerous health records—headaches, menstrual cycle notes, diet information, and so on—you may prefer some sort of lined pages that will help you neatly organize the information for fast reference.

Important Medical Information to Note

What kind of medical information and records do you want to maintain in your journal? In Chapter 3, we discussed the types of symptoms your doctor may want you to record in a monthly symptom diary. Most such records include a list, by the day of your menstrual cycle, of symptoms experienced and the severity of those symptoms (usually noted as mild, moderate, or severe). Some typical symptoms included in symptom diaries or calendars are mood swings, irritability, insomnia, weight change, headache, increased appetite, fatigue, depression, and forgetfulness. When you're preparing to begin your menopause journal, talk to your doctor to find out what symptoms he or she would most like for you to track over the next few months.

Though your menopause journal is much more than just this list of physical and emotional symptoms, those records are an important source of information for both you and your doctor, so choose them carefully. Here are some ideas:

Keep a diet journal: List the foods you eat, serving sizes, and calorie counts if you're concerned about tracking the source of weight gain you may be experiencing or improving your nutrition. Many women have no idea how much they eat during the day, or how well their diet conforms to the recommendations set forward by most health experts. (See Chapter 13 for more information on those guidelines.) You may keep this as a separate journal, and you may keep it for a period of a few months only, depending upon your goals for the record. If you're trying to lose weight, you may want to list your weekly weigh-in results with your diet record.

Keep an exercise journal: When you note the type of exercise you do each day, the length of time you exercise, number of repetitions, and related information, you'll be able to track your progress and note any associations between your exercise, your symptoms, weight changes, and overall feelings of well-being. This record can help encourage you to upgrade your exercise plan to keep it challenging and effective as your body's strength and endurance improve. The record also can give you—over time—an idea of which types of exercise seem to work best for you.

Track all cyclical symptoms: Many women experience cyclical symptoms as they move through perimenopause. For example, hot flashes, migraine headaches, or insomnia may occur at specific points in the menstrual cycles. Your symptom calendar will help you track these recurring symptoms. But you should also be certain to note days in which you have extraordinary feelings of calm, optimism, or energy. Don't just be on high alert for negative days, track those positive feelings as well. Your "up" days may occur on a regular basis, and could provide you and your doctor with important information about hormone cycles, diet, or other factors that contribute to them.

Note changes in medication or supplements: You don't need to begin each day's journal entry with a list of all of the vitamins and routine medications you've taken on that day; one entry in your journal should include that list, for the record. But note any changes from your daily routine; add and remove medications as your prescriptions change or end, and note changes in the types or amounts of vitamin and mineral supplements you're taking. If you switch from brand-name prescriptions to generic, record that, too. If you forget to take any of your daily medications or supplements, or run out of your supply temporarily, make sure that you note that—even if you have to go back later and add the information.

FACTS

Tracking your diet is also a helpful way to uncover connections between the foods you eat and menopause symptoms. You may discover that certain foods contribute to fatigue, hot flashes, headaches, or insomnia. This is just one example of how your journal can offer important information about overall patterns of habits and symptoms that may occur during your menopause passage.

Finding Time to Write

Let's face it; your biggest challenge in writing a journal may not be choosing a format or deciding what kinds of information you most want to record. Beginning the habit of writing a journal is the most important part of the process, and it can be the most difficult, as well. If you fail to keep your journal regularly, it loses much (but not all) of its value as a record of change; if you don't know where you've been, it's harder to understand where you may be going. Keeping a daily journal is a habit worth acquiring, however, so here are some ideas to help you in that effort:

Try to write at least once a day: If you can't bring yourself to note all of the items you think you should, at least write something. Like most worthwhile endeavors, journaling takes practice.

If time is a problem, "automate" as much as possible: Find ways to create spreadsheets, checklists, or other time-saving formats so you can note items quickly that don't need a great deal of description. (You can preprint daily diet lists, or—if your doctor doesn't have a preprinted symptom list or diary—devise your own shorthand system for noting symptoms.) If one form of journaling seems to be too time-consuming, and you're tempted to stop, just try a different form. You're new at this, so you may not find your best method with your first attempt.

Begin by writing at the same time and in the same place every day: Over time, you may choose to be freer in your approach to journaling, but when you're just getting started, setting a regular schedule may help you develop the journaling habit.

Try timed practice: If you have a hard time writing about your feelings in your journal, try some timed exercises. Write whatever comes into your head for ten to twenty minutes for three days in a row; you can describe the smell of a cup of coffee, your memories of your first kiss, a particularly nasty encounter you had at work that day, or reflections on your drive home. This kind of free writing can teach you to record your thoughts and open up to the writing process.

Appendix A
Glossary

AMENORRHEA. a cessation or absence of menstrual periods.

ANDROGENS. male hormones normally produced in small quantities by the female ovaries and adrenal glands, with the greatest quantities occurring at the midpoint of a woman's menstrual cycle. Androgens are thought to promote a healthy sex drive and are sometimes prescribed as part of a full regimen of hormone replacement therapy.

ANDROPAUSE. *See* **MALE MENOPAUSE.**

ANGINA. a squeezing, heaviness, or tightness in your chest that happens when your heart muscle is deprived of oxygen.

ANTIOXIDANTS. certain vitamins, including vitamins A, C, E, and beta carotene, found in some brightly colored fruits and vegetables, considered to be important tools in warding off heart disease and some cancers and may even reduce age-related macular degeneration (age-related vision loss).

ATHEROSCLEROSIS. a blood vessel condition that develops when the buildup of plaque on arterial walls narrows the arterial passage and thus limits the amount of blood that can flow through the arteries to nourish the heart, brain, kidneys, and other organs.

BIOFEEDBACK. a technique in which individuals are trained to monitor their breathing, heart rate, and blood pressure (with the use of various instruments), then change the rate of those functions through relaxation techniques or visual imagery.

BIOFLAVONOIDS. naturally occurring plant substances found in many brightly colored fruits and vegetables, such as cherries, oranges, other citrus, grapes, leafy vegetables, wine, and some types of red clover. Bioflavonoids are being studied for the treatment of a number of conditions, including the control of bleeding, hemorrhoids, and varicose veins.

BMI (BODY MASS INDEX). a measurement of a person's percentage of fat, determined by dividing a person's weight by their height.

CALCITONIN. a hormone produced by the parathyroid gland to help regulate calcium levels in the bloodstream, and in so doing, protect bone density. Calcitonin is available in prescription form for the treatment of postmenopausal osteoporosis.

CARDIOVASCULAR DISEASE. a term used to describe a variety of heart diseases, illnesses, and events that impact the heart and circulatory system, including high blood pressure and coronary artery disease.

CHEMOTHERAPY. the use of potent medications to treat cancer, usually by affecting cells that are rapidly growing, such as the cancer cells themselves.

CORONARY ARTERY DISEASE. a common form of heart disease that results when the heart receives inadequate amounts of oxygen-rich blood through its arteries. This disease usually occurs when arteries become lined with heavy deposits of plaque—a substance made up of fat and calcium in a condition known as atherosclerosis.

DENDRITES. the fine appendages at the ends of brain cells that transmit brain signals.

DEHYDROEPIANDROSTERONE (DHEA). an important hormone in the female body that decreases as a woman ages and declines dramatically after menopause. DHEA is thought to combat memory and bone loss, and it may help to maintain breast and cardiovascular health.

DHEA. *See* **DEHYDROEPIANDROSTERONE.**

ENDOMETRIAL CANCER. cancer of the endometrium.

ENDOMETRIAL HYPERPLASIA. a precancerous condition of the endometrium that is typically diagnosed through a biopsy or sampling of the uterine lining, a procedure most doctors perform in their office.

ENDOMETRIUM. the lining of the uterus.

ENDORPHINS. naturally occurring substances released by the brain that resemble opiates, and are considered to be the brain chemicals that make you feel happy and content.

ESTRADIOL. the main form of estrogen produced by the ovaries, and the body's most efficient and potent estrogen.

ESTROGEN. a sex hormone produced by the ovaries, pituitary gland, and (in small quantities) by body fat. During puberty, estrogen stimulates the development of adult sex organs and the adult female breasts, hips, and buttocks. Estrogen helps to retain calcium in bones, regulates the balance of **HDL** and **LDL CHOLESTEROL** in the bloodstream, and aids the maintenance of blood sugar level, memory functions, and emotional balance.

FIBROIDS. benign growths of muscle cells that develop within or on the uterine wall.

FOLLICLE STIMULATING HORMONE (FSH). produced by the pituitary gland, promotes follicle development within the ovary, thus allowing certain eggs to mature and the follicle cells surrounding each egg to produce estrogen in preparation for fertilization.

FSH. *See* **FOLLICLE STIMULATING HORMONE.**

HDL CHOLESTEROL. the high-density lipoprotein fraction of cholesterol ("good" cholesterol) that helps prevent heart disease by breaking up and carrying the low-density lipoprotein (LDL cholesterol) out of the bloodstream and into the liver for metabolism and evacuation in the feces.

HEART PALPITATIONS. the uncomfortable sensation that the heart is beating rapidly, out of sequence, too strenuously, or in some other abnormal fashion.

HIPPOCAMPUS. the part of the brain responsible for creating, storing, and retrieving memory.

HORMONE REPLACEMENT THERAPY (HRT). therapy consisting of estrogen or a combination of estrogen and progestin designed to replace the loss of these hormones in menopause and thus combat the effects of this deficiency, including bone loss, vaginal atrophy, hot flashes, and other conditions.

HOT FLASHES (FLUSHES). hot flashes or flushes can be mild or severe, but in general, they involve a fast-spreading sensation of warmth through the face, neck, and shoulders. Hot flashes are the result of fluctuating hormone levels, but their triggers, intensity, and frequency vary from woman to woman. Hot flashes that occur during sleep are often known as **NIGHT SWEATS**.

HRT. *See* **HORMONE REPLACEMENT THERAPY.**

HYPERTENSION. high blood pressure that occurs when arteries become too inflexible to allow an ample supply of blood to circulate, especially under periods of exertion or stress, thus causing excess pressure against arterial walls.

Severe or ongoing high blood pressure can lead to stroke and other life-threatening conditions.

HYSTERECTOMY. the surgical removal of the uterus that may or may not also be accompanied by the removal of the cervix and/or ovaries. If ovaries remain, the hysterectomy doesn't necessarily cause menopause, though menstrual bleeding ceases.

INDUCED MENOPAUSE. a cessation of menstrual cycles that occurs when a woman has her ovaries surgically removed in a procedure called **OOPHORECTOMY**, or when a woman's ovaries cease to function prematurely as a result of medication, radiation, a lack of nutrition, or excessive exercise. With treatment and intervention, some nonsurgical types of induced menopause may be temporary. *See also* **TEMPORARY MENOPAUSE.**

INSOMNIA. an inability to fall and/or remain asleep that occurs three or more nights a week.

ISOFLAVONES. a type of plant estrogen found in soybeans, red clover, and (in much lower quantities) green tea, peas, pinto beans, lentils, and other legumes, that may have benefits in treating some symptoms of menopause.

KEGEL EXERCISE. an exercise designed to strengthen the muscles of the pelvic floor to improve vaginal muscle tone, improve sexual response, and limit involuntary urine release due to **STRESS URINARY INCONTINENCE**.

LDL CHOLESTEROL. Low-density lipoprotein cholesterol ("bad" cholesterol) is the fraction of total cholesterol that accumulates as fat deposits (plaques) on arterial walls.

LH. *See* **LUTEINIZING HORMONE.**

LUTEINIZING HORMONE (LH). a hormone produced by the pituitary gland, LH has multiple functions, one of which is prompting ovulation.

MAJOR DEPRESSION. an emotional disorder characterized by extreme or prolonged feelings of sadness, despair, guilt, or hopelessness so debilitating that they affect one's normal quality of life and/or work performance.

MALE MENOPAUSE. known as **ANDROPAUSE** to the medical community, male menopause is associated with an age-related decrease in male hormone levels in men; symptoms can include lethargy, depression, mood swings, insomnia, hot flashes, irritability, and decreased sexual desire and function.

MAMMOGRAM. a low-dose X-ray of the breast used to screen for or examine lumps that may signify breast cancer.

MENARCHE. the first menstrual period.

MENOPAUSE. the permanent end of menstruation and fertility. *See also* **NATURAL MENOPAUSE, INDUCED MENOPAUSE,** *and* **TEMPORARY MENOPAUSE.**

MIGRAINE HEADACHES. intensely painful headaches thought to be associated with spasms in constricted blood vessels in the brain. Women who suffer migraines describe them as pounding headaches that can produce nausea, vomiting, and a painful sensitivity to light, noise, and odors.

NATURAL MENOPAUSE. the cessation of all periods resulting from the halt of ovarian hormone production that is spontaneous and not the result of other physical or pathological conditions or treatments; natural menopause is diagnosed when a women has had twelve months of **AMENORRHEA**.

NIGHT SWEATS. *See* **HOT FLASHES.**

NUTRACEUTICALS. though no legally determined or internationally accepted definition exists for this term, in the marketplace the term is used to describe foods or dietary supplements that claim to deliver some sort of medication or compound designed to offer a specific medical benefit.

OBESITY. a condition of being more than 30 percent over your ideal weight, or having a **BODY MASS INDEX (BMI)** of 25 or higher.

OMEGA-3 FATTY ACIDS. essential fatty acids found in fish, nuts, flaxseed, tofu, and in soybean and canola oils, that help nourish the hair and nails, and offer a number of benefits for cardiovascular health.

OOPHORECTOMY. the surgical removal of one or both ovaries.

OSTEOPOROSIS. a chronic disease in which a loss of bone mass results in porous, fragile bone that is prone to fracture. An age-related disease in menopause, osteoporosis can manifest itself sooner in women who have risk factors.

OVULATION. The release of a mature egg from a properly developed ovarian follicle.

PAP SMEAR. a tissue sample taken (as a swab) during an internal vaginal exam to test for precancerous cell changes and cervical cancer.

PERIMENOPAUSE. the period of transition to natural menopause during which the body undergoes endocrinologic and biologic changes resulting from declining ovarian hormone production; symptoms can include irregular menstrual periods, hot flashes, vaginal dryness, insomnia, and mood swings. Perimenopause can last up to six years (four years is average) and ends after twelve months of **AMENORRHEA**.

PHYTOHORMONES. natural substances found in some herbs and other plants that may help to regulate plant growth. Some types, referred to as phytoestrogens, can bind to the human body's estrogen receptors and may act like an estrogen or an antiestrogen on the body, depending upon their particular type and dosage.

PMDD. *See* **PREMENSTRUAL DYSPHORIC DISORDER.**

PMS. *See* **PREMENSTRUAL SYNDROME.**

POLYP, UTERINE. small, tag-shaped growths of uterine tissue, attached to the lining of the uterus. Polyps can cause irregular bleeding; doctors remove them to confirm there is no precancerous change.

PREMENSTRUAL DYSPHORIC DISORDER (PMDD). a debilitating type of premenstrual syndrome that can include symptoms such as severe depression, anxiety, sleep disturbances, and fatigue in addition to a wide range of physical disturbances. Though **PREMENSTRUAL SYNDROME (PMS)** and PMDD differ in severity, diagnosis, and treatment, both seem to be linked to the way the body processes and responds to reproductive hormones and possibly serotonin.

PREMENSTRUAL SYNDROME (PMS). a condition occurring ten to fourteen days before the onset of menstrual bleeding and involving physical and emotional symptoms that include bloating, water retention, pelvic pressure or cramping, headaches or migraines, irritability, mood swings, difficulty concentrating, and food cravings.

PROGESTERONE. a female sex hormone, produced in largest amounts during and after **OVULATION** that prepares the uterus for the implantation of a fertilized egg.

PROGESTIN. a chemical name for various types of synthetic progesterone. Progestin is used in **HRT** to balance the effects of estrogen on the **ENDOMETRIUM** and prevent endometrial hyperplasia and cancer.

SELECTIVE ESTROGEN RECEPTOR MODULATORS. a class of drugs used to help prevent bone loss. Raloxifene is one example of a **SERM**.

SERM. *See* **SELECTIVE ESTROGEN RECEPTOR MODULATORS.**

STATINS. cholesterol-lowering drugs.

STRESS URINARY INCONTINENCE. the unpredictable and involuntary loss of urine caused by weakened sphincter muscles (the muscles that surround the urethra) and often triggered by an event such as a sneeze or cough.

TEMPORARY MENOPAUSE. an interruption of the ovarian function that prevents the production of hormones that accompany the maturation and release of oocytes (eggs). Temporary menopause can follow chemical or radiation therapies or result from excessive exercise, weight loss, or inadequate nutrition. *See also* **INDUCED MENOPAUSE**. When the contributing condition stops, ovulation and menstruation begin again.

TRIGLYCERIDES. a type of fat found in the blood; other types of this fat include butter, margarine, and vegetable oil. Triglyceride levels are checked in total fasting lipid-profiles (blood tests, sometimes called coronary panels, that check levels of **HDL** cholesterol, **LDL** cholesterol, and triglycerides).

URETHRA. the external opening in the bladder through which the body releases urine.

URGE INCONTINENCE. involuntary bladder spasms that can be triggered by the sight, sound, or even thought of water or urination; the sudden reflex need to urinate causes the spasm and an accompanying release of urine.

URINARY TRACT INFECTIONS (UTI). a bladder infection due to bacteria that typically has entered the bladder through the urethra through the process of intercourse, improper wiping techniques, poor hygiene, or other reasons.

UTI. *See* **URINARY TRACT INFECTIONS.**

VAGINAL ATROPHY. a condition characterized by the drying and shrinking of the vaginal lining. As the body's estrogen production diminishes with menopause, the vagina produces fewer secretions, so the vaginal wall becomes less lubricated and flexible and more prone to tears and cracking.

VAGINITIS. an infection due to bacteria, yeast, or other pathogens, resulting in discomfort, itching, and/or abnormal discharge.

VASOMOTOR SYMPTOMS. hot flashes or night sweats that result from hormonal fluctuations in menopause and perimenopause.

APPENDIX B

References and Resources

Print and Online Articles, Journals, and Magazines

American College of Obstetricians and Gynecologists. "A Healthy Diet." ACOG Patient Education pamphlet number AP151, ACOG, Washington, D.C.

American Council on Exercise. "Don't Deprive Yourself of the Rewards of Exercise." The American Council on Exercise Fit Facts, online, *www.acefitness.org*.

American Heart Association. "Risk Factors and Coronary Heart Disease." American Heart Association Scientific Position, November 26, 2001.

Association of Reproductive Health Professionals. "Mature Sexuality: Disorders of Desire and Alternative Approaches." ARHP Clinical Proceedings, electronic edition, December, 1999, online, *www.arhp.org/clinical/cp12-99/cp12992.htm*

Association of Reproductive Health Professionals. "Perimenopause Update." ARHP Clinical Proceedings, electronic edition, August, 2000, online, *www.arhp.org/CPAugust_2000/perimenopause_update.htm*

Bakos, Susan Crain. "From Lib to Libido: How Women Are Reinventing Sex for Grownups," Modern Maturity Magazine, Sept./Oct., 1999.

Brzezinski, Amnon, et al. "Short-Term Effects of Phytoestrogen-Rich Diet on Postmenopausal Women." *Menopause: The Journal of the North American Menopause Society* 4, no. 2 (1997): 89–94.

Carandang, Jennifer, et al. "Recognizing and Managing Depression in Women throughout the Stages of Life." *Cleveland Clinic Journal of Medicine*, 67, no. 5 (2000): 329–338.

Carpenter, Siri. "Does Estrogen Protect Memory?" by Siri Carpenter, *Monitor on Psychology* 32, no. 1 (2001).

"Estrogen Lifts Mood in the Perimenopause," Women's Health Weekly News, reprinted in *Health & Sexuality*, Winter 2001.

Fisher, Linda. AARP/Modern Maturity Sexual Survey conducted by NFO Research, Inc. Washington, D.C.: AARP, 1999.

Guthrie, Janet R. and Lorraine Dennerstreing. "Weight Gain, Somatic Symptoms, and the Menopause." *Menopausal Medicine* 9, no. 3 (2001).

"Health for Life," a special issue of *Newsweek* magazine, Fall/Winter 2001.

Holman, Marcia. "Managing the Lesser-Known Effects of Estrogen Loss." MedscapeHealth, online, *www.health.medscape.com*.

Jacobs Institute of Women's Health Expert Panel on Menopause Counseling "Guidelines for Counseling Women on the Management of Menopause." Jacobs Institute of Women's Health, online, *www.jiwh.org*.

Kahn, David A., et al. "Depression during the Transition to Menopause: A Guide for Patients and Families," in Expert Consensus Guideline Series, A Postgraduate Medicine Special Report. New York: The McGraw-Hill Companies, Inc., 2001.

Krauss, Ronald M. "Diet and Cardioprotection: Sorting Fact From Fiction." *Menopause Management* 11, no. 1 (2002).

Kurtzweil, Paula. "Lessening the Pressure: Array of Drugs Tames Hypertension." *FDA Consumer Magazine*, July–August 1999.

Mayo Foundation for Medical Education and Research. "Headline Watch: New Evidence of ERT Risks," online, *www.MayoClinic.com*, March 23, 2001.

McNagny, Sally E., et al. "Personal Use of Postmenopausal Hormone Replacement Therapy by Women Physicians in the United States." *Annals of Internal Medicine* 127 (1997): 1093–1096.

"Menopause." On The Alternative Medicine Channel, a member of HealthCommunities.com, online, *www.alternativemedicinechannel.com*.

Menopause Guidebook. Cleveland, OH: North American Menopause Society, 2001.

Murphy, Penelope, ed. *The American College of Obstetricians and Gynecologists Guide to Managing Menopause*. Washington, D.C.: ACOG, 2001.

Newton, K. M., et al. "Women's Beliefs and Decisions About Hormone Replacement Therapy." *Journal of Women's Health* 6 (1997): 459–65.

"Physical Activity and Health: A Report of the Surgeon General." Center for Disease Control online fact sheet, *www.cdc.gov.*

"The Role of Isoflavones in Menopausal Health." Consensus Opinion of the North American Menopause Society. *Menopause: The Journal of the North American Menopause Society* 7, no. 4 (2000): 214–229.

Ryan-Haddad, Ann and Nasrin Piri. "What Options Exist for Postmenopausal Breast Cancer Survivors with Hot Flashes?" U.S. Pharmacist 24, no. 9 (1999).

Scheiber, Michael D., et al. "Dietary Inclusion of Whole Soy Foods Results in Significant Reductions in Clinical Risk Factors for Osteoporosis and Cardiovascular Disease in Normal Postmenopausal Women." *Menopause: The Journal of the North American Menopause Society* 8, no. 5 (2001): 384–392.

Smyth, J., et al. "Effects of Writing about Stressful Experiences on Symptom Reduction in Patients with Asthma or Rheumatoid Arthritis." *Journal of the American Medical Association* 281 (1999): 1304–1309.

"Stealing Time," notes on the film by John Rubin and Ann Tarrant, PBS Online, *www.PBS.org.*

Still, Christopher D. "Health Benefits of Modest Weight Loss." Healthology Press, online, *www.ABCNews.com.*

Takanishi, Gayle C. "Drug Therapies for Hot Flashes in Breast Cancer Survivors." *Women's Health in Primary Care* 3, no. 11 (2000).

"Therapeutic Options During Perimenopause and Beyond." Section G of the Menopause Core Curriculum Study Guide, presented by the North American Menopause Society.

"Too Hot to Handle: Sex and Women over Fifty," in *Vitality: Health and Wellness for Midlife and Beyond*, online, *www.menopausehealth.com.*

Utian, Wolf H. and Pamela P. Boggs. "The North American Menopause Society 1998 Menopause Survey. Part I: Postmenopausal Women's Perceptions about Menopause and Midlife." *Menopause: The Journal of the North American Menopause Society* 6, no. 2 (1999): 122–128.

Weinstein, Sheryl. "New Attitudes Towards Menopause." *FDA Consumer Magazine*, March, 1997 (revised February, 1998).

"What Is Perimenopause," on Menopause Online, *www.menopause-online.com.*

Wyon, Y., et al. "Effects of Acupuncture on Climacteric Vasomotor Symptoms, Quality of Life, and Urinary Excretion of Neuropeptides among Postmenopausal Women." *Menopause: The Journal of the North American Menopause Society* 2, no. 1 (1950): 3–12.

Other Books on Menopause and Women's Health

Allison, Kathleen Cahill. *The American Medical Association Complete Guide to Women's Health.* New York: Random House, Inc., 1996.

DeAngelis, Lissa and Molly Siple. *Recipes for Change.* New York: Dutton Books, 1996.

Goldstein, Steven R. and Laurie Ashner. *The Estrogen Alternative.* New York: G.P. Putnam and Sons, 1998.

Greer, Germaine. *The Change: Women, Aging, and the Menopause.* New York: Alfred A. Knopf, 1992.

Moquette-Magee, Elaine. *Eat Well for a Healthy Menopause.* New York: John Wiley and Sons, Inc., 1996.

Northrup, Christiane. *The Wisdom of Menopause: Creating Physical and Emotional Health and Healing During the Change.* New York: Bantam Doubleday Dell, 2001.

Sheehy, Gail. *The Silent Passage*: Menopause, rev. ed. Random House, 1998.

Professional Organizations and Informational Resources

The American Association of Retired Persons (AARP)
601 E Street NW
Washington, D.C. 20049
www.aarp.org

The American Cancer Society
800-ACS-2345
www.cancer.org

American College of Obstetricians and Gynecologists (ACOG)
409 12th Street SW
Washington, D.C. 20024-2188
202-638-5577
www.acog.org

American Diabetes Association
1701 North Beauregard Street
Alexandria, VA 22311
800-342-2383
www.diabetes.org

The American Heart Association
7272 Greenville Avenue
Dallas, TX 75231
800-AHA-USA1
www.americanheart.org

The American Lung Association
1740 Broadway
New York, NY 10019
800-LUNG-USA
www.lungusa.org

The American Menopause Foundation
350 Fifth Avenue, Suite 2822

New York, NY 10119
212-714-2398
www.americanmenopause.org

The American Psychiatric Association
1400 K Street NW
Washington, D.C. 20005
888-357-7924
www.psych.org

The Association of Reproductive Health Professionals (ARHP)
2401 Pennsylvania Avenue NW, Suite 350
Washington, D.C. 20037
800-804-7374
www.arhp.org

Food and Nutrition Information Center Agricultural Research Service, USDA
National Agricultural Library, Room 105
10301 Baltimore Avenue
Beltsville, MD 20705-2351
301-504-5719
www.nal.usda.gov/fnic

Help for Incontinent People (HIP)
P.O. Box 544
Union, SC 29379
800-BLADDER

The National Cancer Institute
Bldg. 31, Room 10A31
31 Center Drive, MSC 2580
Bethesda, MD 20892-2580
800-4-CANCER
www.nci.nih.gov

The National Center for Complementary and Alternative Medicine (NCCAM)
NCCAM Clearinghouse
P.O. Box 7923
Gaithersburg, Maryland 20898
Toll Free: 888-644-6226
International Telephone: 301-519-3153
E-mail: *info@nccam.nig.gov*

National Institute of Diabetes and Digestive and Kidney Diseases (NIDDK)
NIDDK, NIH, Building 31, Room 9A04
31 Center Drive, MSC 2560
Bethesda, MD 20892-2560
www.niddk.nih.gov

National Menopause Foundation
800-MENO-ASK

National Osteoporosis Foundation
1232 22nd Street NW
Washington, D.C. 20037-1292
202-223-2226
www.nof.org

The National Sleep Foundation
1522 K Street NW, Suite 500
Washington, D.C. 20005
202-347-3471
www.sleepfoundation.org

The North American Menopause Society
P.O. Box 94572
Cleveland, OH 44101
440-442-7550
www.menopause.org

Index

THE EVERYTHING ANTI-AGING BOOK

By Donald Vaughan

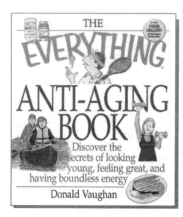

Containing the most up-to-date anti-aging research available, *The Everything® Anti-Aging Book* is the essential resource for both the young in body and the young at heart. It explains the aging process in simple terms, and details the many methods of slowing down natural aging to improve physical and mental health and quality of life. Packed with tips on everything from nutrition and exercise to spirituality and herbal remedies, this easy-to-follow reference teaches you how to age healthfully and gracefully.

Trade paperback, $12.95
1-58062-565-7, 304 pages

OTHER *EVERYTHING®* BOOKS BY ADAMS MEDIA CORPORATION

Everything® **After College Book**
$12.95, 1-55850-847-3

Everything® **American History Book**
$12.95, 1-58062-531-2

Everything® **Angels Book**
$12.95, 1-58062-398-0

Everything® **Anti-Aging Book**
$12.95, 1-58062-565-7

Everything® **Astrology Book**
$14.95, 1-58062-062-0

Everything® **Astronomy Book**
$14.95, 1-58062-723-4

Everything® **Baby Names Book**
$12.95, 1-55850-655-1

Everything® **Baby Shower Book**
$12.95, 1-58062-305-0

Everything® **Baby's First Food Book**
$12.95, 1-58062-512-6

Everything® **Baby's First Year Book**
$12.95, 1-58062-581-9

Everything® **Barbecue Cookbook**
$14.95, 1-58062-316-6

Everything® **Bartender's Book**
$9.95, 1-55850-536-9

Everything® **Bedtime Story Book**
$12.95, 1-58062-147-3

Everything® **Bible Stories Book**
$14.95, 1-58062-547-9

Everything® **Bicycle Book**
$12.00, 1-55850-706-X

Everything® **Breastfeeding Book**
$12.95, 1-58062-582-7

Everything® **Budgeting Book**
$14.95, 1-58062-786-2

Everything® **Build Your Own Home Page Book**
$12.95, 1-58062-339-5

Everything® **Business Planning Book**
$12.95, 1-58062-491-X

Everything® **Candlemaking Book**
$12.95, 1-58062-623-8

Everything® **Car Care Book**
$14.95, 1-58062-732-3

Everything® **Casino Gambling Book**
$12.95, 1-55850-762-0

Everything® **Cat Book**
$12.95, 1-55850-710-8

Everything® **Chocolate Cookbook**
$12.95, 1-58062-405-7

Everything® **Christmas Book**
$15.00, 1-55850-697-7

Everything® **Civil War Book**
$12.95, 1-58062-366-2

Everything® **Classical Mythology Book**
$12.95, 1-58062-653-X

Everything® **Coaching & Mentoring Book**
$14.95, 1-58062-730-7

Everything® **Collectibles Book**
$12.95, 1-58062-645-9

Everything® **College Survival Book**
$14.95, 1-55850-720-5

Everything® **Computer Book**
$12.95, 1-58062-401-4

Everything® **Cookbook**
$14.95, 1-58062-400-6

Everything® **Cover Letter Book**
$14.95, 1-58062-312-3

Everything® **Creative Writing Book**
$14.95, 1-58062-647-5

Everything® **Crossword and Puzzle Book**
$14.95, 1-55850-764-7

Everything® **Dating Book**
$12.95, 1-58062-185-6

Everything® **Dessert Cookbook**
$12.95, 1-55850-717-5

Everything® **Diabetes Cookbook**
$14.95, 1-58062-691-2

Everything® **Dieting Book**
$14.95, 1-58062-663-7

Everything® **Digital Photography Book**
$12.95, 1-58062-574-6

Everything® **Dog Book**
$12.95, 1-58062-144-9

Everything® **Dog Training and Tricks Book**
$14.95, 1-58062-666-1

Everything® **Dreams Book**
$12.95, 1-55850-806-6

Everything® **Etiquette Book**
$12.95, 1-55850-807-4

Everything® **Fairy Tales Book**
$12.95, 1-58062-546-0

Everything® **Family Tree Book**
$12.95, 1-55850-763-9

Everything® **Feng Shui Book**
$14.95, 1-58062-587-8

Everything® **Fly-Fishing Book**
$12.95, 1-58062-148-1

Everything® **Games Book**
$12.95, 1-55850-643-0

Everything® **Get-A-Job Book**
$12.95, 1-58062-223-2

Everything® **Get Out of Debt Book**
$12.95, 1-58062-588-6

Everything® **Get Published Book**
$12.95, 1-58062-315-8

Everything® **Get Ready for Baby Book**
$12.95, 1-55850-844-9

Everything® **Get Rich Book**
$12.95, 1-58062-670-X

Everything® **Ghost Book**
$14.95, 1-58062-533-9

Everything® **Golf Book**
$12.95, 1-55850-814-7

Everything® **Grammar and Style Book**
$12.95, 1-58062-573-8

Everything® **Great Thinkers Book**
$14.95, 1-58062-662-9

Everything® **Travel Guide to
    The Disneyland Resort®,
    California Adventure®,
    Universal Studios®, and
    Anaheim**
$14.95, 1-58062-742-0

Everything® **Guide to Las Vegas**
$12.95, 1-58062-438-3

Everything® **Guide to New England**
$14.95, 1-58062-589-4

Everything® **Guide to New York City**
$12.95, 1-58062-314-X

Everything® **Travel Guide to Walt Disney
    World®, Universal Studios®, and
    Greater Orlando, 3rd Edition**
$14.95, 1-58062-743-9

Everything® **Guide to Washington D.C.**
$12.95, 1-58062-313-1

Everything® **Guide to Writing
    Children's Books**
$14.95, 1-58062-785-4

Everything® **Guitar Book**
$14.95, 1-58062-555-X

Everything® **Herbal Remedies Book**
$12.95, 1-58062-331-X

Everything® **Home-Based Business Book**
$12.95, 1-58062-364-6

Everything® **Homebuying Book**
$12.95, 1-58062-074-4

Everything® **Homeselling Book**
$12.95, 1-58062-304-2

Everything® **Horse Book**
$12.95, 1-58062-564-9

Everything® **Hot Careers Book**
$12.95, 1-58062-486-3

Everything® **Hypnosis Book**
$14.95, 1-58062-737-4

Everything® **Internet Book**
$12.95, 1-58062-073-6

Everything® **Investing Book**
$12.95, 1-58062-149-X

Everything® **Jewish Wedding Book**
$14.95, 1-55850-801-5

Everything® **Judaism Book**
$14.95, 1-58062-728-5

Everything® **Job Interview Book**
$12.95, 1-58062-493-6

Everything® **Knitting Book**
$14.95, 1-58062-727-7

Everything® **Lawn Care Book**
$12.95, 1-58062-487-1

Everything® **Leadership Book**
$12.95, 1-58062-513-4

Everything® **Learning French Book**
$12.95, 1-58062-649-1

Everything® **Learning Italian Book**
$14.95, 1-58062-724-2

Everything® **Learning Spanish Book**
$12.95, 1-58062-575-4

Everything® **Low-Carb Cookbook**
$14.95, 1-58062-784-6

Everything® **Low-Fat High-Flavor
    Cookbook**
$12.95, 1-55850-802-3

Everything® **Magic Book**
$14.95, 1-58062-418-9

Everything® **Managing People Book**
$12.95, 1-58062-577-0

Everything® **Meditation Book**
$14.95, 1-58062-665-3

Everything® **Menopause Book**
$14.95, 1-58062-741-2

Everything® **Microsoft® Word 2000 Book**
$12.95, 1-58062-306-9

Everything® **Money Book**
$12.95, 1-58062-145-7

Everything® **Mother Goose Book**
$12.95, 1-58062-490-1

Everything® **Motorcycle Book**
$12.95, 1-58062-554-1

Everything® **Mutual Funds Book**
$12.95, 1-58062-419-7

Everything® **Network Marketing Book**
$14.95, 1-58062-736-6

Everything® **Numerology Book**
$14.95, 1-58062-700-5

Everything® **One-Pot Cookbook**
$12.95, 1-58062-186-4

Everything® **Online Business Book**
$12.95, 1-58062-320-4

Everything® **Online Genealogy Book**
$12.95, 1-58062-402-2

Everything® **Online Investing Book**
$12.95, 1-58062-338-7

Everything® **Online Job Search Book**
$12.95, 1-58062-365-4

Everything® **Organize Your Home Book**
$12.95, 1-58062-617-3

Everything® **Pasta Book**
$12.95, 1-55850-719-1

Everything® **Philosophy Book**
$12.95, 1-58062-644-0

Everything® **Pilates Book**
$14.95, 1-58062-738-2

Everything® **Playing Piano and
    Keyboards Book**
$12.95, 1-58062-651-3

Everything® **Potty Training Book**
$14.95, 1-58062-740-4

Everything® **Pregnancy Book**
$14.95, 1-58062-146-5

Everything® **Pregnancy Organizer**
$15.00, 1-58062-336-0

Everything® **Project Management Book**
$12.95, 1-58062-583-5

Everything® **Puppy Book**
$12.95, 1-58062-576-2

Everything® **Quick Meals Cookbook**
$14.95, 1-58062-488-X

Everything® **Resume Book**
$12.95, 1-58062-311-5

Everything® **Romance Book**
$12.95, 1-58062-566-5

Everything® **Running Book**
$12.95, 1-58062-618-1

Everything® **Sailing Book, 2nd Ed.**
$12.95, 1-58062-671-8

Everything® **Saints Book**
$12.95, 1-58062-534-7

Everything® **Scrapbooking Book**
$14.95, 1-58062-729-3

Everything® **Selling Book**
$12.95, 1-58062-319-0

Everything® **Shakespeare Book**
$14.95, 1-58062-591-6

Everything® **Slow Cooker Cookbook**
$14.95, 1-58062-667-X

Everything® **Soup Cookbook**
$14.95, 1-58062-556-8

Everything® **Spells and Charms Book**
$12.95, 1-58062-532-0

Everything® **Start Your Own Business Book**
$14.95, 1-58062-650-5

Everything® **Stress Management Book**
$14.95, 1-58062-578-9

Everything® **Study Book**
$12.95, 1-55850-615-2

Everything® **T'ai Chi and QiGong Book**
$12.95, 1-58062-646-7

Everything® **Tall Tales, Legends, and Other Outrageous Lies Book**
$12.95, 1-58062-514-2

Everything® **Tarot Book**
$12.95, 1-58062-191-0

Everything® **Thai Cookbook**
$14.95, 1-58062-733-1

Everything® **Time Management Book**
$12.95, 1-58062-492-8

Everything® **Toasts Book**
$12.95, 1-58062-189-9

Everything® **Toddler Book**
$14.95, 1-58062-592-4

Everything® **Total Fitness Book**
$12.95, 1-58062-318-2

Everything® **Trivia Book**
$12.95, 1-58062-143-0

Everything® **Tropical Fish Book**
$12.95, 1-58062-343-3

Everything® **Vegetarian Cookbook**
$12.95, 1-58062-640-8

Everything® **Vitamins, Minerals, and Nutritional Supplements Book**
$12.95, 1-58062-496-0

Everything® **Weather Book**
$14.95, 1-58062-668-8

Everything® **Wedding Book, 2nd Ed.**
$14.95, 1-58062-190-2

Everything® **Wedding Checklist**
$7.95, 1-58062-456-1

Everything® **Wedding Etiquette Book**
$7.95, 1-58062-454-5

Everything® **Wedding Organizer**
$15.00, 1-55850-828-7

Everything® **Wedding Shower Book**
$7.95, 1-58062-188-0

Everything® **Wedding Vows Book**
$7.95, 1-58062-455-3

Everything® **Weddings on a Budget Book**
$9.95, 1-58062-782-X

Everything® **Weight Training Book**
$14.95, 1-58062-593-2

Everything® **Wicca and Witchcraft Book**
$14.95, 1-58062-725-0

Everything® **Wine Book**
$12.95, 1-55850-808-2

Everything® **World War II Book**
$14.95, 1-58062-572-X

Everything® **World's Religions Book**
$14.95, 1-58062-648-3

Everything® **Yoga Book**
$14.95, 1-58062-594-0

*Prices subject to change without notice.

EVERYTHING KID'S SERIES!

Everything® **Kids' Baseball Book, 2nd Ed.**
$6.95, 1-58062-688-2

Everything® **Kids' Cookbook**
$6.95, 1-58062-658-0

Everything® **Kids' Joke Book**
$6.95, 1-58062-686-6

Everything® **Kids' Mazes Book**
$6.95, 1-58062-558-4

Everything® **Kids' Money Book**
$6.95, 1-58062-685-8

Everything® **Kids' Monsters Book**
$6.95, 1-58062-657-2

Everything® **Kids' Nature Book**
$6.95, 1-58062-684-X

Everything® **Kids' Puzzle Book**
$6.95, 1-58062-687-4

Everything® **Kids' Science Experiments Book**
$6.95, 1-58062-557-6

Everything® **Kids' Soccer Book**
$6.95, 1-58062-642-4

Everything® **Kids' Travel Activity Book**
$6.95, 1-58062-641-6

Available wherever books are sold!
To order, call 800-872-5627, or visit us at everything.com

Everything® is a registered trademark of Adams Media Corporation.